NURSING WOUNDS

NURSING WOUNDS

*Nurse Practitioners, Doctors,
Women Patients and the
Negotiation of Meaning*

SUE FISHER

Rutgers University Press • New Brunswick, New Jersey

Library of Congress Cataloging-in-Publication Data

Fisher, Sue, 1936–
    Nursing wounds : nurse practitioners, doctors, women patients, and the negotiation of meaning /
Sue Fisher.
        p.   cm.
    Includes bibliographical references.
    ISBN 0-8135-2180-7 (cloth). — ISBN 0-8135-2181-5 (pbk.)
    1. Nurse practitioner and patient.   2. Physician and patient.   3. Women patients.
    4. Women—Health and hygiene—Sociological aspects.   5. Interpersonal communication.   I. Title.
    [DNLM: 1. Nurse-Patient Relations.   2. Physician-Patient   Relations.   3. Women.
    4. Communication.   WY 87 F536n 1995]
    RT82.8.F56   1995
    610.69'6—dc20
    DNLM/DLC
    for Library of Congress   94-46485
                                    CIP

British Cataloging-in-Publication information available

CONTENTS

ACKNOWLEDGMENTS

Although the writing of this book was an individual project, I was extremely lucky to be in a fertile environment. My thinking was shaped by the work of feminist and critical scholars who came before me, and I was also enriched by the Monday night lectures at the Center for the Humanities and by my semester spent as a faculty fellow there. Not only does the Center provide an opportunity to hear academics whose work is at the cutting edge of intellectual thought, but, in the best scholarly tradition, it facilitates discussion and, thus, learning. In addition, I was supported by a generous sabbatical system, which provided the time needed to think, read, and grow, and by the generosity of colleagues. Mary Ann Clawson and Joe Rouse were never too busy to read my work, give me comments, and introduce me to the work of others who they thought would be helpful. And Ann duCille provided the title I had been searching for. I owe her a special debt.

I am also indebted to the undergraduate students whose comments have, over time, contributed immensely to this project. Some of these students took the course "Discourse, Text, and Gender" and worked with fresh eyes on the doctor–patient and nurse practitioner–patient transcripts. Some came to talk about their own projects. In either case, they provided stimulating insights and interesting topics for further exploration. Most notable among these students were Lisa Nash, Karen Turk, and Jen Langdon.

There were others—both academic and not—whose support was essential. To protect their confidentiality, I cannot thank by name the doctors, nurse practitioners, and patients who allowed me to observe and record their interactions. I can, however, thank some of the many friends whose enthusiasm for this project was a constant. Most notable among them are Kathy Davis, Joann Falbo, Nina Gregg, Elizabeth Isele, Peggy Myers, and Ann Louise Shapiro.

I also owe a special debt to my sons, who believed in me before I believed in myself; to my special friend and colleague Alexandra Todd, who made the early years both fun and growthful and whose continued friendship and support have been invaluable; to Irene Spinnler and Connie Colangelo, who made sure all the commas were in place and helped to get the book ready for publication; and to my long-time editor, Marlie Wasserman, who encouraged and supported me during my early days as a scholar and has since become a valued friend.

Thank you all!

NURSING WOUNDS

ONE

NURSES DO IT BETTER

In 1985, on a bright, sunny day late in December, I was having lunch with two friends who were nurse practitioners. One was a part-time administrator and the other a part-time clinician; both taught in a community-health program of a college of nursing in a major northeastern university, and both were committed to nursing education, especially to the education of clinically trained nurse practitioners.[1]

The conversation at lunch that day changed the direction of my research. I had just finished a book manuscript that analyzes the way doctors—obstetricians/gynecologists and family-practice physicians—deliver health care.[2] The research took more than six years—years spent in examining rooms observing and recording how health care is delivered to women and talking with caregivers about the ways they communicate with patients, principally women patients.

I explained to my luncheon companions that I was disheartened, disillusioned, and more than a little bit concerned. I could not imagine myself in another examining room observing the oppressive ways doctors provide health care to women. I could no longer envision trying to teach uninterested medical students and residents how to listen and communicate effectively. I was a medical sociologist interested in the delivery of health care to women, and I was burnt out.

It was excruciating to be a mainly silent observer, as I had been, watching how physicians encouraged women patients to have medical procedures that were not warranted on strictly medical grounds, to have unnecessary hysterectomies, while not encouraging them to have diagnostic procedures that were both cost-effective and medically sound, to have regular Pap smears (Fisher 1986). It was equally painful to continue my participation in the education of residents. It was frustrating to realize that my impact on medical students, residents, and their attending staff physicians was, at best, minimal.

I was a social scientist working in a medical-science setting with an almost exclusively male population. Where they were interested in learning about the science of medicine and gaining experience in clinical practice, I talked about the art of medicine, about social psychological skills. More specifically, I talked about the ways providers communicate with women patients and the impact their communication practices have on the delivery of health care—a topic that, unfortunately, was all too easily classified as unimportant and was dismissed. While I was disqualified by my topic and by my interest in women, neither my gender nor the nature of my professional expertise helped. Residents accepted the all-male attending medical staff as appropriate teachers, while I was a woman and a social scientist committed to improving the ways health care was delivered to women. In this context, it was not surprising to feel that my influence had been inconsequential and, given the time and energy I expended, to feel frustrated.

It was also frightening to learn how little power even a well-informed woman patient had. I had documented the communication strategies through which doctors "sell" women treatments they do not need and fail to encourage them to have diagnostic procedures that might be beneficial. I also saw that on rare occasions patients could intervene by asking questions and could thereby change the diagnostic and treatment processes (Fisher 1986). Personally and politically these successes gave me hope. I hoped that women who were well informed about medical facts and about the subtleties of communication could gain some control in the management of their own health care.

When I was diagnosed with just the kind of medical problem I had been studying, it was a terrible shock to learn that in the face of a potentially life-threatening condition my information was no protection. As an exceptionally well-informed patient, I wanted to participate and pressed to do so. While I chose my issues carefully, I nevertheless found myself in a double bind. Good patients are compliant; however, compliant patients all too often receive health care that is not in their best interest. I knew the costs associated with unquestioned acceptance of medical definitions. I learned firsthand the costs associated with trying to intervene in the diagnosis and treatment. My desire to be fully informed and to participate in decisions about my health care was seen as confrontational. Patients who confront and challenge their doctors are not compliant, and frequently the price they pay for their failure to conform is a high one. I still carry the medical injury that was the punishment for my inappropriate behavior.[3]

My luncheon companions listened sympathetically. Then they asked a question that redirected my research interests. They asked whether I had considered studying the ways nurse practitioners deliver health care. They enthusiastically explained that beginning in the mid-1960s and in response to a critical shortage of doctors, nursing first developed a certificate program and later master's and Ph.D. degrees for nurses with advanced training in physical assessment.[4] To the tradition of a caring nurse, these practitioners added the technical skill and medical knowledge of a primary-care provider. Specifically, they added the ability to take medical histories, perform physical examinations, make diagnoses, recommend treatments, manage acute care, and stabilize chronic illnesses. According to the nurses I was lunching with, in becoming medically well-trained primary-care providers who were equally well versed in social psychological skills, nurses were able to deliver care better than doctors.

While their enthusiasm for the training, efficiency, and effectiveness of nurse practitioners was boundless, they were all too well aware of the political problems facing the nursing profession. Nurses had long been subordinate to doctors, who not only had a monopoly over the practice of medicine but also had tremendous political clout. In this context it was difficult to establish the status of nurse practitioners as autonomous professionals—a difficulty well documented both in nursing history and in current struggles.

The research project from which this book developed was born in the conversation that day. As a feminist, I found the thought that nurses do it better an appealing one. I liked the idea that they nursed wounds better, that they cured the physical body and cared for more socioemotional concerns as well. However, to pose a system that adds caring to curing as the justification for this claim seemed quite problematic, as were the suggestions that caring could provide the authorization for nurse practitioners' quest for professional autonomy, the ground for their professional identity as health-care providers, and the basis for a different kind of provider-patient relationship.

As a concept, caring has embedded in it some of the deepest dimensions of traditional gender differentiation in our society (Toronto 1989). Historically, it has participated in the reinscription of two convergent sets of social relations. It has reinforced a sexual division of labor and women's participation in a secondary labor market; and it has fortified what some refer to as the public patriarchy (Brown 1981). To name caring, then, as the ground for a different kind of clinical practice and the basis of increased professional status runs the risk of reinscribing the very social relations nursing is resisting.

In addition, medical sociologists have long suggested that better social psychological skills would improve the medical relationship. If doctors encouraged patients to talk about the social context of their lives, if they empowered patients by maximizing their voices, then the asymmetry so typical in the medical relationship could be minimized. However, even in research on the doctor-patient relationship, this is an open empirical question, and nursing research is even more ambiguous. Although quantitative studies support nurse practitioners' claims that they have excellent social psychological skills and are as medically competent as primary-care physicians, there is almost no qualitative empirical information that describes in detail their actual performance in examining rooms. Without this kind of data, we have no way of knowing what nurse practitioners' social psychological skills look like in the day-to-day clinical practice of nursing.

Similarly, while a substantial body of data documents that the doctor-patient relationship is overwhelmingly characterized by its asymmetrical nature, there is much less agreement about how to form theories about the seemingly persistent nature of this relationship. Thus, for nursing to equate caring with social psychological skills and to imply that it has the potential to remedy the all-too-persistent asymmetry in the medical relationship raises important questions with interesting policy ramifications. If nursing predicates its struggle for professional status on caring, if nurses care and doctors do not, is caring a gendered activity performed only by women or only in a profession gendered female? Is curing, then, the "real" stuff and caring the something special women can add? If so, the gendered nature of caring in all probability would limit its applicability.

Since medicine remains both male-defined and predominantly male in its makeup, it is unlikely that as a gendered activity caring would be incorporated into the routine practice of medicine. From this perspective a team approach to the delivery of care seems more reasonable than the professional autonomy that nursing seeks.[5] However, a team that has doctors doing the curing with nurses helping out as physician extenders while also performing their unique, gendered-linked activity of caring not only recirculates traditional gender and professional relationships but also limits potential policy recommendations.

HISTORICAL, EMPIRICAL, AND THEORETICAL NARRATIVES

In addressing these issues—issues that are political, empirical, and theoretical in nature—I begin by telling several interrelated stories: a gender story about caring as a historical concept, a qualitative empirical story about how caring translates into clinical practice and professional status, and a theoretical story about caring as a remedy for the asymmetrical encounter all too characteristic of the doctor-patient relationship. At a time when the health-care system in the United States is in crisis, when a majority of the American people say they want a change, and when even the President is talking about the need to transform the way we deliver medical care in this country, these stories help us to understand why nursing staked its claim to professional autonomy on such a fragile concept as caring as well as to ascertain whether medicine and nursing provide essentially different sites for the delivery of care.

To determine whether nurses care for women patients' physical and social psychological wounds differently, I continue with a detailed empirical description that compares the ways doctors and nurse practitioners deliver health care. I then move on to discuss how theory can help make sense of the differences and similarities I found. And I end by suggesting how both empirical findings and theoretical conclusions might be useful in the policy-making process.[6]

The Gendered Story: Caring as a Historical Concept

Caring, at least since the emergence of the "cult of domesticity" (Cott 1977), has been gendered. In rapidly changing times it has played an important role in shoring up the ideology of gender difference. As the informal, unpaid labor that women do to protect and promote the well-being of others, as a routine feature of the domestic economy, as a part of women's everyday life in the family and in the community, caring contributes to the glorification of the home and women's roles in it. There has been, in addition, a strong association between caring and taking care of, including taking care of the health of others. Women have long been responsible for providing the domestic conditions necessary for both the maintenance of health and the recovery from illness (Graham 1985).

In the social transformation from preindustrial to modern industrial work patterns, women began to turn their usual domestic occupations into paid work (Cott 1977). Health care was no exception. In her history of American nursing, Reverby (1987) argues that caring for the needs of others for love became, for some, caring for others as paid labor.[7] In the early years paid nursing was a trade "professed" in the market place, learned at home and practiced by older women with no formal training or schooling. When nursing moved out of the home and into the hospital and especially after the Nightingale-based reforms, female character built on the obligation to care contributed to the sacrifice of autonomy on what Reverby (1987:200) refers to as "the altar of altruism."

Caring has remained central to nursing. The later separation of nursing education from nursing service did not diminish either the obligation to care or nursing's position as a woman's occupation. Neither a university education nor the move toward professional autonomy eliminated the cultural identification of nursing with caring—an identification evident in the ways nurse practitioners as emerging health-care professionals used caring to support their claims to both clinical expertise and professional status.

During the 1960s, when federal policies in the United States were directed toward countering societal inequalities, including inequalities in health care, a new health professional came into being—the nurse practitioner. While nurses had long been subordinate to physicians by custom and law (Melosh 1982), nurse practitioners sought to establish themselves as fellow professionals; however, they had problems doing so.[8] The medical profession has "an official approved monopoly to the right to define health and illness and to treat illness" (Freidson 1970:5)—a right based in its control over a body of medical knowledge and technical skill as well as in its freedom from outside control, its professional autonomy. If nurse practitioners share a body of medical knowledge and technical skills with physicians and if they are positioned in relationship to them as physician extenders, on what could their professional autonomy rest?

To make a place for themselves, nurse practitioners turned caring from an obligation into a virtue. By operationalizing it as psychosocial skills and as patient education and prevention, they could depict caring both as the basis for a different kind of clinical practice and as a special kind of knowledge and skill, which they could control. At first glance, nurse practitioners' contention that they add caring to curing does not seem to be an empty assertion. An ample literature based on quantitative studies supports the claim that nurse practitioners provide health care that is comparable to the care provided by primary-care physicians—care that is of high quality, efficient, effective, and economical (Lynaugh and Fagin 1988, Shamansky 1985, Diers and Molde 1979, Sacket et al. 1974). In addition, nurse practitioners are generally acclaimed for their psychosocial skills (Lohr and Brooks 1984). It is this combination of medical and psychosocial skills that is said to differentiate nursing from medical practice and that grounds nurse practitioners' claim for professional autonomy.

Caring, couched in terms of qualities understood as natural—qualities that could jump from the private to the public sphere without threatening the identity of their bearer—has been vital to important transitions for women. While remaining pivotal to women's identity, caring took women from the home to nursing in the paid labor force. At a later time, when women's participation in the public sphere as nurses working in a secondary labor market was more accepted, caring emerged as central to another battle. Caring has been at the heart of the campaign to move from being a doctor's handmaiden (Melosh 1982) to being an autonomous medical practitioner. Moreover, it grounds the identities of nurse practitioners as women, providing the conceptual basis for both a new political reality—the nurse practitioner as autonomous medical provider—and a different kind of provider-patient relationship, one that integrates medical and psychosocial skills. Yet, when all is said and done, little qualitative data describe in detail what nurse practitioners actually do in examining rooms.

The Empirical Story: Caring as Clinical Practice

Overwhelmingly, researchers, myself among them, have concentrated on the doctor-patient relationship. We have gathered an impressive array of empirical materials suggesting that the medical relationship is characterized by an asymmetry between provider and patient and by an almost exclusive concern with medical topics to the nearly total exclusion of the social and biographical contexts of patients' lives (Todd 1989, Mishler 1984). This medical relationship rests on the medical model, which presents illness as the organic pathology of individual patients. Within this perspective neither nonorganic complaints nor the social context of patients' lives fits comfortably. The medical problem to be solved is located in the individual's body—organs malfunction in mechanistic style. Diagnosis identifies the specific etiology—the specific pathological disturbance—and treatment optimally returns the system to its normal state of balance.

The system of care nursing claims to offer challenges this model. Nurse practitioners argue that the problems patients bring to examining rooms cannot be separated from the complex social and psychological lives they lead. A nursing practice that integrates the social psychological and the medical aspects of care, that nurses wounds holistically, blurs the distinction between the medical and the social, the physiological and the psychological.

Since the delivery of health care is essentially a communication event, this challenge to the medical model implies skills that are linguistically based. To gain access to biographical information, nurse practitioners have to encourage patients to speak about their lives. But the suggestion that patients be encouraged to disclose the social and biographical contexts of their lives—a practice said to minimize the asymmetry of the provider-patient relationship and to maximize the patient's voice—raises empirical questions without ready answers. Does a nursing practice that adds caring to curing truly minimize the asymmetry so characteristic of the provider-patient relationship? And, in so doing, does it maximize the patient's voice by adding the social to the medical, which characterizes doctor–patient communication? If so, does it provide a discourse upon which to redefine the medical model and the clinical practice that flows from it? These questions ask what a nursing practice that adds caring to curing looks like and whether it provides the basis for a different kind of provider-patient relationship. There are additional questions about whether differences in communication style have any influence on medical outcomes or social understandings.

But to date we lack the kind of information that would allow us to answer any of these questions. Without such data, we do not know how caring or, for that matter, quality and effectiveness translate into nursing practice. Nor can we understand what consequences, if any, such translations might have. It is one thing to posit that nurse practitioners offer a system of care; it is quite another to display what this system of care looks like in practice.

The Theoretical Story: Caring as a Remedy

At another level the ways we understand the relationships between provider and patient, the medical and the social, and medicine and society pose theoretical issues—issues central to sociological studies by Mishler (1984), Silverman (1987), and Waitzkin (1983). While these studies focus on the doctor-patient relationship, the issues they raise are directly applicable to the nurse practitioner–patient relationship.

Mishler (1984) describes the practice of medicine as being divided into two separate discourses—the voice of medicine and the voice of the "lifeworld." Doctors, who are oriented almost exclusively to the technical, bioscientific aspects of medicine, have the dominant voice, the voice of medicine, while patients, who are subordinate, have difficulty inserting their voice, the voice of the lifeworld. Reformers, like Mishler, challenge the dominance of the medical model and call for a more humanistic, patient-centered medical practice that includes both social psychological and medical aspects of patients' lives.

From this perspective, if patients are treated as whole people rather than sick body parts, if the medical and social, the pathological and the psychological are valued equally, if the emphasis on diagnosis and treatment is extended to include education and prevention, if patients are recognized as experts on their own lives, if doctors ask open-ended questions, if they share medical information, if they listen to what patients have to tell them, and if they encourage patients to participate, then an asymmetrical relationship could become more egalitarian. Providers could maximize the patient's voice by broadening the medical model, by having a humanistic attitude, and by minimizing their power and sharing their knowledge. These changes would enable patients to participate in the diagnostic and treatment processes and thereby enhance their potential for agency.

Silverman (1987) is critical of Mishler's remedy to the problems in the medical encounter. He argues that Mishler's call to humanize medical practice by encouraging patients to speak about their lives relies on faulty assumptions. It poses the social in opposition to the medical, assuming that doctors speak in the medical and patients speak in the social voice. Encouraging a "discourse of the social" (Silverman, 1987:191) as an authentic (it speaks the truth) voice is presented by Mishler as inevitably liberating; and calling for and inciting this voice, then, could correct the imbalances in the medical relationship. Mishler's recommendation, what Silverman refers to as his call for a discourse of the social, sounds much like the system of care nurse practitioners claim to provide. But, rather than relying on polarities such as social/lifeworld and medical/biological, Silverman suggests that we see in the medical consultation a plurality of voices, each interrupting and interpenetrating the other. Doctors and patients can and do speak in both medical and social voices.

Speaking in a common language, they create a field of power that governs them both.

Waitzkin (1983) is also critical of the kind of reforms Mishler suggests, but he has a different conception of how power works than Silverman does. For him, doctors and patients do not speak in a common voice. They do not form a field of power that governs them both. Nor does the voluntary inclusion of a humanistic discourse of the social resolve the troubles in the medical relationship. To Waitzkin, both positions present the medical relationship as if it were independent of the larger social context; both accept the context of patients' lives uncritically. Since the medical relationship does not occur in a vacuum, larger social contradictions penetrate the purported intimacy of the medical consultation. During medical encounters doctors routinely do ideological work that reflects and reinforces dominant structural arrangements, especially economic arrangements, encouraging patients' consent to them. Both social and medical discourses, then, are deeply political.

For Waitzkin, the remedy is for socially conscious doctors to engage in ideological work that reveals and resists oppressive structural arrangements. The starting place for social change is a new form of medical practice that redirects patients toward political action. Doctors can help patients break the ideological chains that bind them.

What we have here is the kind of theoretical debate that characterizes most academic endeavors. Mishler contends that if doctors solicit and pay attention to the voice of the patient's lifeworld, the medical relationship will be improved. By contrast, for Silverman medical and social voices are not distinct. A field of power develops to govern both doctor and patient, who speak a common language with medical and social voices interrupting and interpenetrating each other. In addition, since power does not flow in one direction from doctors to patients, Silverman is also positioning himself in opposition to more materialist accounts like Waitzkin's. For Waitzkin, the practice of medicine, whether spoken in the voice of medicine or the voice of the lifeworld, reflects and reinforces larger structural arrangements—arrangements that socially conscious doctors can encourage patients to resist.

With its professed system of care nursing seems an ideal site for exploring these conflicting positions. Not only do nurses claim to add caring to curing, but caring appears to be defined in ways that index just the kinds of social psychological skills Mishler is calling for.

DO NURSES DO IT BETTER?

The claim that nurse practitioners provide a system of care raises questions with important ramifications. Empirically we do not know what nurse practitioners actually do in examining rooms, how caring translates into clinical practice. And theoretically we do not know whether caring can remedy the problems all too characteristically associated with the doctor-patient relationship. Without this information, we have no principled way to decide whether we should adopt a policy that continues to support a team approach to the delivery of care. While it can be argued that a team approach positions the doctor as a fatherlike, dominant member and the nurse as the wifelike, subordinate helper—albeit a helper with special caring skills—and in so doing reproduces both gendered and professional meanings, there is little basis for policy recommendations that could alter this situation. If we had the missing information, perhaps we could argue for policies that would support the professional autonomy of nonphysician providers and broaden the scope of their practice without reinforcing the sexual division of labor or women's participation in a secondary labor market. In the Epilogue I make such an argument.

Against the background of Mishler's (1984) call for a discourse of the social and Silverman's (1987) and Waitzkin's (1983) different theoretical stance, I present detailed empirical analyses of four consultations—two with family-practice doctors and two with nurse practitioners. By juxtaposing the ways nurse practitioners and doctors communicate with women patients during medical encounters, we can garner evidence that sheds light on empirical questions about what nurse practitioners actually do in examining rooms—about caring as medical practice—and on theoretical questions about the viability of caring as a discourse of the social that remedies the problems in the provider-patient encounter. In turn, this information suggests a direction for future policy, which I discuss in both Chapter Eight and the Epilogue.

Gathering this information is a necessary first step; making sense out of it analytically is the next problem. If I find that nurses do it better, how will I account for this finding? Will I maintain that the social or biological nature of women's lives predisposes them to perform in ways that are both different from and better than the ways men perform? Or will I claim that the differences between doctors and nurses are to be found in their different educational experiences? For many researchers, including myself, neither explanation suffices. We would be equally uncomfortable treating gender as an undifferentiated category of meaning and analyzing an experience lifted out of its specific social and historical context.

KNOWLEDGE SEEKING AND KNOWLEDGE MAKING

Finding my way out of the dilemma posed by the claim that nurses do it better requires an epistemological shift—a shift that is influenced by feminist theorizing about the nature of reality and the production of knowledge. Haraway (1991), Harding (1991), and Fraser (1989) each argue that knowledge seeking and knowledge making are situated practices.[9] Fraser (1989:7), for example, does what she calls "situated theorizing." She situates herself in the knowledge-seeking and knowledge-making process. While I discuss the reasoning behind this epistemological shift in Chapter Two, these formulations about the production of knowledge guide my research process as well as the plan of the book, and so I want to address them here.

As a knowledge seeker, I can use situated theorizing to ground my analysis, to present myself and the knowledge I am making as an active perceptual process, an embodied objectivity. I am, after all, a white, middle-aged, middle-class, professional woman. I am a feminist, an academic, and a medical sociologist with a long history of social activism. From these embodied positions I frame research problems and gather, discuss, and analyze data. In the end, from these locations I will contribute to the collection of situated knowledges.

Once I locate myself in this way, it is easy to understand my strong commitment to changing the organization of the health-care system in the United States, improving the delivery of care to women, and bettering women's status as caregivers—commitments that drew me to this project and have shaped it. It is just a short step to move from my own embodied position to the institutional location of doctors and nurse practitioners and to question their status as knowledge makers. Here again I am indebted to Fraser (1989). While she explores how social welfare institutions have provided an implicit but nevertheless powerful interpretive grid of "normative, differently valued gender roles and gendered needs" (9), and I examine how meanings are produced in the institutions of medicine and nursing, we both treat these institutions as sites for situated theorizing. And, in so doing, we both probe to see how "institutionalized patterns of interpretation" (9) function to reproduce or undermine hegemonic understandings.

The Research Process: Knowledge Seeking

I started this project by speaking to the women I already knew at the college of nursing who had interested me in the way nurse practitioners deliver care in the first place. They invited me to speak to their colleagues in the community-health section of the nurse-practitioner training program in their college. When we met, my first task was to listen to their problems. I wanted to learn both how these nurse practitioners saw the practice of medicine as well as where and how my research might be useful to them.

In an interesting and informative discussion they explained that, like most of the faculty in this school of nursing, they divided their time between teaching and clinical practice. From this dual location, they were all too aware of the problems nurse practitioners faced in the examining room and professionally, problems they then shared with me. The patients in their clinical practice usually were those in need of health care but locked out of the system—the poor, the underinsured and the uninsured, the old, and those who were chronically ill, often with multiple illnesses. Compared with doctors, they were underpaid and frequently denied the privileges doctors routinely enjoyed, which many were fighting for.

All across the United States in state-by-state struggles, nurse practitioners were engaging in a battle for the right to write and sign prescriptions (prescriptive privileges), the right to admit patients into hospitals and to supervise their care once admitted (hospital privileges), and the ability to be paid directly by a third party for services rendered.[10] The battle lines were clearly drawn. While nurse practitioners were struggling to become autonomous medical providers, the established forces in medicine were fighting to keep them in their proper places as members of a team in which the doctor retains authority and the nurse, no matter how defined (also see note 5), remains a glorified handmaiden (Melosh 1982).

While in some states some nurse practitioners had won some privileges, the battles were hardly over. Quite the contrary. As the number of primary-care doctors multiplied and competition between these providers and nurse practitioners grew, the pressure increased to limit the scope of nursing practice; this pressure was reflected in medical journals, as discussions about the differences between nursing and medical practice escalated. The implication in these articles was always the same: for better health care, why settle for less—nurses—when you could have more—real doctors? These same issues underlay lawsuits in which nurse practitioners were charged with practicing medicine without a license.

After listening to the nurse practitioners, I spoke about the research I wanted to do and explained how I thought it might be useful in future political battles. It would provide qualitative empirical data heretofore missing in the literature on nursing. Given that there was a lot of information about what doctors do in examining rooms and little about what nurse practitioners do, information about what nurse practitioners actually do and how it is the same or different from what doctors do might be put to good political use in the battles against the institutional and structural forces currently constraining nurse practitioners' ability to practice autonomously. I then asked to be invited into their examining rooms, where I would watch and audiotape their interactions with patients and the ways they nursed patients' wounds.

At first only one nurse practitioner stepped forward. She said, "Sure! Come watch me." I did. Word spread that it was neither invasive nor threatening to have me in the examining room, and there were benefits. I provided good, often helpful feedback about the interactional dynamics of the provider-patient relationship. Others volunteered.

Each nurse practitioner who agreed to participate signed an

informed-consent form. Before I went into examining rooms, the nurse practitioners asked the patients whether they would participate in a study. When patients agreed, I explained the study and presented the informed consent for them to sign. Only after these forms were signed did I begin to observe. Over the next three years I observed seven nurse practitioners as they provided health care at three different sites—an indigent care setting associated with a teaching hospital, a neighborhood health clinic in a poor urban area, and an outreach clinic in a suburban area with a large population of older people.[11] I also did in-depth interviews with participating nurse practitioners.

Six of the nurse practitioners were women; five were trained in the same school; two taught in the nursing college and combined their teaching with a clinical practice; six had considerable experience, having practiced for a number of years. All of the nurse practitioners were white and middle-class; they ranged in age from their early thirties to their mid-forties. All, even the male nurse practitioner, identified themselves as feminists, and six out of the seven identified their politics as left of center.[12] In fact, many made a political choice to become nurse practitioners at a time when they could have become doctors. They explained that being a nurse allowed them to care for patients in a way they thought that doctors could not. It also allowed them to have a life in addition to their professional life in a way they believed that doctors did not.

A clinical day is divided into two half-day sessions—a morning and an afternoon clinic. I observed each nurse practitioner for fourteen half-day sessions as they provided care to women and men, old and young, and of a variety of races and ethnicities.[13] Why fourteen? Any number of sessions would have been arbitrary. I chose fourteen and spaced them out over weeks and sometimes months. I wanted my coming and going to seem a normal part of clinic life. I wanted to "hang around" long enough to get a feel for what being a nurse practitioner or a patient in these settings was like. I wanted to observe over a period of time to get a sense of how nurse practitioners provided care individually and collectively—to begin to clarify the interactional patterns that characterize the way they deliver care.

These seven nurse practitioners observed for fourteen half-day sessions each became the subjects for the analysis that follows. After explaining that I wanted to study the ways providers and patients communicated with each other, and with signed consent forms in hand, I audiotaped each encounter. These tapes were transcribed, and I spent hours pouring over them.

I had been aware from the beginning that the nursing encounters I observed felt different from the medical consultations I had studied earlier. One of the first things I noticed was that I often left the examining room feeling that I knew the patient. During the consultation I had learned about her life as well as the specifics of her medical complaint. As I watched I became convinced nurse practitioners were directing interactions in ways that made this knowing possible. I also sensed that both patients' physical and their more social psychological concerns had been dealt with differently. However, there also seemed to be important similarities. Nurse practitioners, like doctors, seemed to direct interactions during consultations and, in so doing, to reproduce the asymmetry found to characterize the medical relationship.

These differences and similarities struck me even more forcefully as I worked with the transcripts. While in the beginning I could not fully articulate what I thought I was seeing, as I studied the transcripts I became better able to document what I had intuitively found. As I moved from one transcript to another, patterns became visible. When I identified a pattern in one transcript, I checked it against the others. Since I knew that in the end I would do a detailed analysis of only a few cases,[14] I wanted to make sure that the cases I picked represented the recurrent patterns I had identified.

I decided to structure the project around a dual comparison. I wanted to know whether the social context of a patient's life was more likely to emerge if the topic under discussion could be identified as social psychological rather than medical in nature and, if so, whether this label structured the provider patient relationship or the ways decisions were reached (or both). To address these questions, I decided to compare the ways doctors and nurse practitioners deliver health care to women patients whose complaints could be easily coded as medical or marked as social psychological. It was my hope that this comparison would display whether medicine and nursing provided different sites for the delivery of care, the production of knowledge, and the negotiation of identity.

I was fortunate. I had just moved to the Northeast from the Southeast, where I had spent the four proceeding years doing research in a model family-medicine practice clinic associated with a teaching hospital. Here white, almost exclusively young, male residents were trained in a setting established to mirror the population and problems in a poor, rural community. The providers, too, mirrored the community. Most were politically conservative. They were from surrounding rural areas in what is euphemistically called the Bible Belt. When their residencies were completed, most would remain in that region.

In this medical setting I also spent considerable time establishing rapport before I began to collect data. I hung around getting to know the providers. I worked with the attending staff to provide training to residents in the social psychological aspects of the delivery of care. Then, with the permission (informed consent) of both providers and patients, I went into examining rooms. I spent hundreds of hours observing and audiotaping forty-three provider-patient consultations.[15] I later had these tapes transcribed. I then analyzed them to find the recurrent patterns and wrote about them (Fisher 1986).

The data gathered in this research setting seemed to provide an ideal contrast to the data I had gathered with nurses. Family-practice physicians and nurse practitioners have much in common.[16] They share a stated commitment to primary care. And they claim to provide patient-centered, holistic medicine that integrates medical and social psychological aspects of health care, just the kind of care that Mishler (1984) and other reformers were calling for, but through separate, and differently gendered, professions.[17] In addition, these professionals were positioned in disparate professional communities and located quite differently in the structural arrangements of society.

I chose the case studies I am about to discuss for their comparability and for their contrasts. After identifying recurrent patterns in the nursing encounters and deciding that I wanted to compare the ways the social gets talked about in provider-patient consultations with complaints that can be easily understood as medical and social, I went back to the transcripts of the doctor-patient encounters I had collected earlier and chose comparable cases. In this way I selected providers, patients, and presenting complaints that were both representative of the larger sample from which they were chosen and closely matched between samples.

However, there were also significant differences. When I discuss medical consultations the doctors I present are men, and when I discuss nursing encounters the nurses are women. This selection represents the populations I observed. Although I spent about four years in the family-medicine practice, only two or three doctors in training during that time were women. The situation with nurse practitioners was even more dire. In the three-year period in which I was doing my research, there were only one or two male nurse practitioners in the area. Thus making these providers the focus of my case studies would hardly have been representative.

While the selection of data for this project can in no way be presented as random, the similarities and differences I discuss in the case studies to follow provide important points of comparison.

The Plan of the Book: Knowledge Making

The first two chapters of the book set the stage for the analysis that follows. This analysis draws on insights in critical and feminist theory that are "simultaneously structural and interpretive" (Fraser 1989:9). In Chapter Two I review feminist scholarship that addresses epistemological assumptions about the justification of knowledge claims. In this work, whether examining the status of reality or the production of knowledge, I propose situated knowledges as a concept capable of bridging earlier either/or positions.

Without a concept like situated knowledges both standpoint (Harding 1986) and constructivist theories provide important insights but also leave significant problems unaddressed (compare Fisher and Davis 1993). In standpoint theories power is characterized as coming from the structural arrangements of society—capitalistic and patriarchal arrangements; however, we are left with penetrating questions about the nature of human agency. In constructivist theories, while power and resistance are portrayed as shared, we are left with no principled way to consider how we might engage in a collective struggle for social change, no basis for contemporary social movements.

This theoretical discussion sets the stage in the later part of Chapter Two for situating the institutions of medicine and nursing in their historical, cultural, and structural contexts. When taken together these theories and the situated discussions of nursing and medicine frame the analysis and conclusions that follow in subsequent chapters. Yet, for some readers, Chapter Two, with its focus on theory and history, may better be left for later reading or be skipped entirely. These readers will be most interested in and engaged by the descriptive materials in Chapters Three through Seven.

In Chapters Three through Six, I explore the knowledge-making practices of providers and patients, addressing two different kinds of complaints—complaints coded as social psychological and those marked as medical. In Chapter Seven I compare the institutions of medicine and nursing as sites for the production of meaning. In each of these chapters I rely on assumptions about "situated embodied knowledges" (Haraway 1991:191)—assumptions I make explicit when I discuss a politics of location in Chapter Eight.

All these chapters take the relationship between the social and the medical as a topic of inquiry, but there are differences. As Mishler (1984), Todd (1989), and others have argued, doctors all too often dismiss the social/biographical contexts of patients' lives as not the "real stuff" of medicine. By bifurcating the medical and the social and treating organic pathology as medical, they leave the way open for two separate but interrelated phenomena. On the one hand, when complaints are diffuse, when they are social or psychological in nature, and when no organic pathology is found, problems are located in patients' heads, not their bodies. These patients are often labeled hypochondriacs, "crocks" in a more clinical lexicon, and treated accordingly. Not only are the social/biographical contexts of their lives ignored, but diagnoses are missed and inappropriate treatments are prescribed (Todd 1989). All too frequently these patients are treated with psychotropic drugs (Prather 1990, Prather and Fidell 1973). Suggestions for remedying these problems include integrating the social context of women's lives by making them legitimate topics of discussion during medical consultations (Todd 1989) and humanizing medical practice by balancing social and medical voices (Mishler 1984).

On the other hand, when complaints are accepted as an indication of organic pathology, it is often assumed that diagnosis and treatment are devoid of the social. In a value-free and objective manner, doctors identify the pathology and treat accordingly. The inclusion of the social context of patients' lives is no more likely with this kind of complaint than with diffuse complaints (Mishler 1984, Todd 1989). In addition, assumptions about the objective nature of medical science obscure the ways that social/ideological factors contribute to both diagnosis and treatment and perpetuate the myth of an objective science as well as the moral and political regressiveness that all too often accompanies it. Here the suggested remedies depend upon exposing medical biases by laying bare the social factors that penetrate the presumed neutrality of a medical diagnosis and recommended treatment. This kind of exposé has been a recurrent topic of feminist and Marxist criticism (Ehrenreich and English 1979, 1973, 1972; Waitzkin 1983).

The discussion that follows addresses these two aspects of the social—the social/biographical and the social/ideological—reformulates them, and explores how the social functions in doctor-patient and nurse practitioner–patient consultations. In Chapters Three and Four, the patients' complaints of nearly passing out and of fatigue are easily coded as social psychological. These encounters, then, seemed to provide an ideal site at which to explore how doctors and nurse practitioners integrate, or fail to integrate, the medical and the social—a site from which to question whether a discourse of the social can maximize the patient's voice and, in so doing, minimize the asymmetry that so often characterizes medical consultations. This discussion also makes visible and explores how social talk fractures into talk about the social/biographical context of patients' lives and into social/ideological talk about how women *should* live their lives.

In Chapters Five and Six, the patients' complaints—vaginal bleeding several years after a hysterectomy and the routine maintenance of diabetes—are just as easily identified as medical. They are, after all, complaints resulting from "real" organic pathology. These consultations, then, seemed to offer a good opportunity to appraise both how the social/biographical is or is not incorporated into medical discussions as well as how social considerations penetrate discussions that are purportedly medical in nature and thereby do ideological work.

Organizing Chapters Three, Four, Five, and Six in this manner risks reiterating the distinctions between the social and the medical inherent in both reformers' remedies and in most Marxist and feminist criticisms and, thus, perpetuating a binary logic that positions the medical and the social as polar opposites. To minimize this risk and to avoid the problems associated with it, in each of these chapters I reposition the analysis. As Silverman (1987) advises, I refigure the medical and the social as discourses that interrupt and interpenetrate each other while also focusing, as Waitzkin (1983) suggests, on how both medical and social discourses do ideological work and are, therefore, deeply political. In the postmodern tradition I treat the transcripts of the doctor–patient and nurse practitioner–patient encounters as texts and scrutinize them by reading against the grain. In so doing, I highlight the ways discourses function to produce knowledge and negotiate identities, illuminating how this knowledge making is different and similar in medical and nursing practices and with complaints marked as social psychological or coded as medical.

In Chapter Seven I switch my analytic gaze from the differences and similarities in the ways doctors and nurse practitioners talk with patients whose complaints are coded as social psychological or marked as medical to how medicine and nursing are institutional sites for the production of meaning. First, I illuminate how the practices of medicine and nursing provide more than health care. They also provide "tacit but powerful interpretive map[s] . . . which can encode and/or undermine sexist and androcentric interpretations . . . erected on the basis of gender-linked dichotomies like domestic versus economic, home versus work, mother versus breadwinner" (Fraser 1989:9) and appropriate versus inappropriate gender and sexual behavior. Second, I illustrate how even though providers and patients do not bring the same resources to their encounters, powerful and institutionally sanctioned interpretations do not go uncontested by patients. Third, I display how neither institutional interpretations nor challenges to them are necessarily homogenous. Doctors, nurse practitioners, and patients do not speak in only one voice. They are each polyvocal, speaking in a plurality of voices that not only interrupt each other but also intersect, compete, and conflict with each other. These voices reproduce contradictory tendencies in the larger society.

The politics of location is the topic of Chapter Eight. Nurse practitioners are women in a gendered profession. As women and as professionals they are located both in a subordinate position to men and a medical profession gendered male and in a superordinate position to other nurses and hospital workers. From my position as an academic feminist simultaneously interested in situated knowledges and committed to changing the ways health care is delivered in the United States, and in the face of today's health-care crisis, it makes good political sense to question whether doctors and nurse practitioners who are situated differently in larger structural and institutional arrangements nurse wounds and, therefore, deliver health care differently. It also makes good political sense to compare how in and through the knowledge-making activities of doctors, nurse practitioners, and women patients professional and gendered identities are produced, dismantled, and transformed.

My goal in this project is to provide a qualitative empirical account of the situated practices through which health care is delivered, knowledge is produced, and identities are negotiated. The information garnered addresses the question I raised earlier about caring as an empirical process. On the basis of this information, I reenter ongoing debates between theoretical positions coded as disparate and address their explanatory power—especially their ability to account for the differences and similarities in the medical and nursing encounters. In so doing I reformulate the theories discussed in this chapter and the next, suggest strategies for nurse practitioners in their battle for professional autonomy, and outline policy recommendations to reorganize the health-care delivery system. These discussions address issues about the organization of the health-care delivery system that have largely been silenced since the medical profession gained its professional monopoly early in the twentieth century.[18]

TWO

SITUATED KNOWLEDGES

Since I first began to work on this project, I have been plagued with questions about how to resolve apparent dichotomies.[1] My first area of concern had to do with the status of reality. Is reality "out there," ready-made, independent of the observer's gaze, just waiting to be discovered? Do the methods of scientific research, then, act as a safeguard such that the discovery of the facts of the real world is an objective, value-free process? Or, by contrast, is reality socially accomplished? Is it part and parcel of what Haraway (1991:185) refers to as the "world-as-code"? In a language-mediated process do social actors produce what passes for reality? Do we as social scientists trace these socially accomplished realities and, in so doing, produce or reproduce them? These questions each capture an accepted way of doing social science research; however, neither more traditional positivistic epistemologies, which Harding (1986) refers to as an empiricist epistemology, nor more radical constructivist ones in themselves satisfy me.

The second issue is closely related to the first and has to do with the relationship between social structure and social action, or structure and meaning. On the one hand, there are theories that locate the power associated with the production of knowledge in the structural arrangements of society. Harding (1986) calls these standpoint theories. On the other hand, there are theories that describe this power as socially constructed. Each of these theories raises different issues. While standpoint theories direct our attention to the ways structural arrangements shape social action and cultural meanings, the focus on human agency, on resistance, is much more limited. By contrast, constructivist theories focus on the ways action and meaning are socially accomplished; however, they have much more difficulty accounting for the structural organization of power. Once again, for me, neither position in itself is convincing. Both standpoint and constructivist explanations limit potential analysis (compare Fisher and Davis 1993).

For example, if I choose a position from the above analytic categories—empiricist or constructivist epistemologies and standpoint or constructivist theories—I can account for how doctors and nurse practitioners provide health care in only two ways. If I find that nurse practitioners practice medicine differently from doctors, I can claim that these differences result from the structural locations of doctors and nurses—their class position, profession, or gender.[2] If they practice medicine similarly, I can argue that these similarities flow directly from the organization of health care. Since by training and experience providers have medical knowledge, technical skill, and power, which patients lack, both nursing and medical practices engender similar asymmetrical arrangements. In either case, I would be relying on a standpoint theory and an empiricist epistemology. Theoretically, the providers' power, their ability to produce meaning, would be produced in a top-down fashion; individual agency would be hard to identify; and resistance would entail escaping from monolithic controls of either a structural or a professional nature (or both). Methodologically, as an objective observer I would locate power as it is enacted in the factual arrangements of the social world.

By contrast, if I abandoned these structural and institutional explanations, I could document the ways doctors, nurse practitioners, and patients construct and deconstruct the reality that is clinical practice and, in so doing, invest it with meaning. Here, I would highlight any similarities and differences I find.[3] I would no longer be relying on a standpoint theory, as power would be socially accomplished; however, in exchange for a view of how actions and meanings are produced, I would lose the ability to locate power structurally. In addition, while in theory I have a choice between methodological positions that place me outside as an objective observer gathering real facts about the social world and those that, while making no truth claims, just offer descriptions of how this world of meaning is produced, in practice this choice is more difficult than it seems. Political and normative assumptions, while not made explicit, are still embedded in the process of making meaning (Harding 1986, 1991; Haraway 1991; Fraser 1989).

This choice between dichotomous positions is troubling not just to me. It is part of an ongoing dialogue with especially important consequences in the philosophy of science and in feminist theory. Epistemological discussions and theoretical developments offer a challenging new analytic option—an option contained in the notion of situated knowledges. I could try to bridge these seemingly contradictory perspectives with an argument that is both more open and more complex.

While still interested in historical, cultural, and structural contexts, I could shift my focus to the ways these arrangements are reproduced and undermined as providers and patients make meaning during the routine activities associated with the delivery of health care. And, in so doing, I could document how in the struggle over dominant and alternative discourses—about women, work, and the nuclear family, about women, age, and sexuality, and about gendered and professional identities—meanings are reinscribed and contested.[4] By treating language as a mediated process in and through which both social action and meaning are accomplished, I would be relying on both standpoint and constructivist theories. And, by analyzing how the production of knowledge—whether by sociologists or by health-care providers—is situated culturally, sociologically, and historically, I could avoid some of the pitfalls of both empiricist and more radical constructivist methodologies. Since this option frames the analysis and conclusions that follow, I will discuss it in some depth.

KNOWLEDGE FROM NOWHERE AND EVERYWHERE

Harding (1991:141) argues that the idea that science identifies and allows the telling of "one true story" presents scientific knowledge seeking as a voice from nowhere. Since there is a direct correspondence between the social world that is out there and its representation, this voice speaks just what it has discovered, taking no responsibility either for the discovery or for any consequences that flow from it.[5] Haraway (1991:189) calls this the "God trick." A voice from nowhere, or the God trick, is possible only if the self and the perceiving mind of the observer are defended in a fortresslike fashion against social and political influences. From this perspective knowledge seeking is devoid of power and knowledge seekers are devoid of responsibility for the knowledge they produce.

While this empiricist epistemology is policed by philosophers, codified by methodological canons, and enshrined by scientists and social scientists alike, in practice even scientists do not act purely on the basis of a disembodied objectivity (Latour and Woolgar 1979). Increasingly since the publication of *The Structure of Scientific Revolutions* (Kuhn 1962), this position has come under attack. It is claimed that the belief in one true story obscures the many ways this story is defined by and is useful to the dominant group, which is Western, bourgeois, patriarchal (Harding 1986). One true story not only advances the self-interest of the elite but also reinforces the status, prestige, and power of the scientist and social scientist. As Rouse (1987) argues, two related points must be made here: one true story obscures the ways that knowledge seeking is already saturated with political interests, values, and desires; and, perhaps even more important, it mystifies the ways power is produced along with knowledge.

If knowledge and power are so intimately intertwined, it makes little sense to claim that objectivity is advanced only by the elimination of all political values—that knowledge comes from nowhere. But if the pursuit of knowledge is not value-free, impartial, and dispassionate, then what are the principles that guide the gathering of evidence and that direct the arguments that support or refute particular positions? Traditionally we are left with what Harding (1991:139) refers to as "judgmental relativism." Either we assume that there are many claims to knowledge and that what seems reasonable to one group might not be to another—a kind of historical, sociological, or cultural relativism. Or we have no principled way to argue against the position that each person's judgment is equally valid—a kind of epistemological relativism that brings us full circle. From this perspective, then, knowledge comes from everywhere.

As Haraway (1991) points out, in the strong constructivist position argued for both in many social studies of science and by many feminists, there are no rational or scientific grounds for making judgments about competing claims. Natural and social worlds are crafted into objects of knowledge. History is a story. Science and social science are contestable texts and fields of power. Here, there is no privileged researcher's perspective, no single story that speaks the truth. Instead, there are power moves. In the production of knowledge, language-mediated actors engage in powerful social practices, and these practices are persuasion.

While this constructivist position goes beyond the prior distinction between good science and bad science, beyond the use and misuse of science (Arditte, Brennan, and Cavarak 1980), and provides good tools for illustrating the contestability of scientific and social scientific constructions, it does not describe a reality from which feminists—activists and academics alike—can take on the reality presented by dominant image makers. Although both Harding (1991) and Haraway (1991) agree that moral and political regressiveness follows from a value-free standard for objectivity, neither is willing to abandon objectivity altogether. Instead, they argue that we need a better account of the world.

Harding and Haraway, along with others, do not want to give up the concept of objectivity but cannot abide the notion of a disembodied objectivity—a gaze from nowhere (Haraway 1991). And they are, in addition, frightened by the inability of radical constructivism to develop rival claims about reality—knowledge from everywhere. Using somewhat different language, they call for an embodied objectivity (Haraway 1991) and a successor science (Harding 1991).

Using the metaphor of vision, Haraway (1991) argues that instead of objectivity as the passive vision associated with positivistic science (in Harding's language, an empirical epistemology), we need an insistent embodiment in which objectivity is readily acknowledged as an active perceptual system that is culturally, sociologically, and historically located. Knowledge seeking, then, would be an active process that simultaneously takes into account the situational contingencies of both knowledge claims and knowing subjects as it engages in a critical practice for recognizing how meanings are made. For Harding (1991), Haraway (1991), and others, it is on this combination of postmodernist accounts of difference and the power of modern critical theories that their commitment to faithful accounts of the real world, rests. These accounts are, for them, about limited locations and situated knowledges.

What is being called for here is a strong concept of reflexivity in which both the researcher and the process of observation cannot be separated from their social context or their social consequences. Researchers would be obligated "to gaze back" (Harding 1991:163) through their theoretical approach and methodological strategies to the historical, sociological, and cultural particularities of their socially situated research projects and to locate themselves in them. In the end we would have a diverse account of reality that would capture what Knorr-Cetina and Cicourel (1981) have called "micro episodes" of interaction as well as more macro social, economic, and political realities. Researchers could then demonstrate how all positions, including their own, comprise privilege and oppression.

Harding and Haraway readily admit that the position they are suggesting is contradictory and leaves many important issues unresolved. For example, we would need to find ways to translate diverse accounts of reality from the perspective of many others located in many different, power-differentiated communities (Haraway 1991) and to define normative standards for choosing among them (Fraser 1989). Nevertheless, our need for strong tools with which to deconstruct the truth claims of hostile scientific and social science research as well as our need for an improved account of reality makes these contradictions necessary and perhaps even constructive.

Harding's (1991) and Haraway's (1991) discussions, while directed primarily toward issues of methodology and epistemology, open up the possibility of addressing how the power associated with the production of knowledge is accounted for—its theoretical adequacy. However, whether the focus is on methodological or on theoretical adequacy, the central task is the same: to question epistemological assumptions about the justification of knowledge claims. In each case, the effort is directed toward correcting partial and distorted versions of traditional analyses.

POWER FROM SOMEWHERE AND EVERYWHERE

Just as the previous methodological discussion fell into two categories—knowledge from nowhere and from everywhere—the theoretical discussion that follows is divided into two sections—power from somewhere and from everywhere. One perspective portrays a monolithic system of control in which power is held by certain groups and exercised from above. Here, power is held by the privileged few. It flows in a top-down fashion from somewhere—from specific locations in the structural arrangements of society. Power, then, is outside of most of us. It impinges upon and socializes us. In feminist versions of this theoretical account, power flows from the structures of patriarchal or capitalist domination or both.

For radical feminists, patriarchy is both a familial and a social system that gives individual men power over individual women, their bodies, their labor, and their children—control that is upheld by men collectively (Brown 1981). While this account refuses to privilege the economy over the ideological conditions of oppression, power is clearly located. It is held by men, individually and collectively, and is exercised from above, shaping women's lives in the process.

Others rely more heavily on Marxism to explain the oppression of women. Even though, as Haraway (1991) reminds us, the modern conception of gender is not found in the writings of Marx and Engels, Marxism has provided important tools for locating power in the structural arrangements of society, especially its economic arrangements, and specifically in the dominant classes. From this perspective, relations between the sexes are a consequence of class relations, and women's subordinate position is related primarily to their participation, or their lack of participation, in the paid labor force.

However, for some, Marxist assumptions about class do not adequately address questions about gender (compare Arditti, Brennan, and Cavarak 1980) or about race. These feminists move to theorize the intersection of class and gender or class, gender, and race. Some call for a dual system of analysis and some for a more unified system,[6] but, however the connections are established, power is located in structures of domination and flows in top-down fashion from them. There are additional core similarities in these positions that have been the subject of much feminist criticism.

First, this top-down argument presents a totalistic vision of power and demonstrates how that power reproduces itself as it shapes both social relations and cultural meanings. Second, these theoretical perspectives, while maintaining that resistance is possible, tend to screen out how those depicted as oppressed contest dominant structural arrangements and culturally hegemonic representations. Escape is defined negatively as "escape from . . . " and is possible if, and only if, women are able to gain control of the oppressive structures that shape their lives and, in so doing, control the definition of themselves and the material conditions of their existence.

Taking several different forms, disputes over the relationship between class and gender or class, gender, and race, capitalism and patriarchy, continue (MacKinnon 1987, Hartsock 1983). Some feminists try to address these criticisms by showing how women resist in the face of structural conditions that restrain them (Gordon 1988, Davis 1988, 1994). Others reject what they refer to as a repressive hypothesis that presents individuals as passive victims of oppressive systems, however these systems are defined (Butler 1990, Riley 1988, Scott 1988). Finding these explanations beyond repair, they have turned to constructivist theories. No longer is power presented as flowing from somewhere—from the structures of capitalist and patriarchal domination. Instead, relying heavily on Michel Foucault, they present power as being everywhere.

Foucault (1979) describes modern forms of power as different from earlier forms.[7] It developed in piecemeal fashion in what he calls "disciplinary institutions" and only later was integrated into larger structural arrangements. By tracking power beyond the economy and by treating the role of intellectuals and experts differently, Foucault (1978, 1979) recasts both the definition of power and its relationship to resistance. At the very center of this position is a vision of power that is neither prohibitive nor repressive. It is instead productive. Power, rather than operating in a top-down fashion through the state, through the economy, or through ideologically based systems of beliefs, operates in a "capillary" fashion, circulating through a multitude of everyday social practices—"micropractices"—that touch people's lives more fundamentally than beliefs.

Here, Foucault is concerned with the processes, procedures, and practices whereby truth/knowledge is produced. These micropractices succeed each other historically and can be uncovered through a method of historical and social description ("genealogy"). Fraser (1989) clarifies how this method operates. A description of the ways power/knowledge functions in particular historical contexts displays how power circulates in and through the production of multiple discourses. Among other things, these discourses produce criteria for truth and falseness and valorize "the institutional licensing of some persons as authorized to offer authoritative knowledge claims and the exclusion of others" (Fraser 1989:20).

If, as Foucault suggests, power no longer flows from somewhere, if it functions in a local, continuous, and productive manner and through numerous everyday micropractices, if it is everywhere and in everyone, and if resistance accompanies power, then the very definition of the political has been expanded. From this perspective, it no longer makes sense to talk about power and resistance as oppositional categories. Power is no longer held by a "clearly identifiable and coherently sovereign group" (Martin 1988:6). Instead, as Rouse (1987:19) points out, "power becomes the mark of knowledge." Similarly, resistance does not occur in a kind of "power free zone" from which one can "just [say] no" to oppression (Fraser 1989:26–27). Instead, there is a politics of everyday life in which power and resistance are produced and dismantled in mundane social practices, especially those occurring in institutional sites such as medicine, education, the family.[8]

Foucauldian postmodernism encourages an analysis of culture as practice—an analysis of multiple sites, situated social practices, and a plurality of agents and discourses crosscutting each other in a complex process. The focus is no longer on the economy or on how systems reproduce themselves. It is, instead, on the situated character of knowledge-production procedures and institutions. But, as Fraser points out, while accounting for the "capillary" character of power, multiple sites of political struggle, and an expanded sense of what counts as political, this perspective provides no way "to consider how all these various struggles might be coordinated and what kinds of change they might accomplish. . . . [They provide] no rhetoric of resistance that could promote the struggles and wishes of contemporary social movements" (Fraser 1989:4).

Like Fraser and others (Haraway 1991, Harding 1991, Bartky 1988, Bordo 1988, Martin 1988), I am attracted to a Foucauldian postmodernism and want to go beyond this interpretive mode to add a structural approach but one that avoids a repressive hypothesis that positions women as passive victims. One way to do this is by accepting the contradictions (Harding 1986, 1991) in different feminist positions. For example, even though radical feminism universalizes women's experience and elevates the patriarchy as its sole ahistorical theoretical justification, it nevertheless directs our attention to the ideological conditions of oppression, making struggles over meaning legitimate topics of analysis (Martin 1988). If this struggle over meaning is located in its historical context, positioned in specific local sites, and if power and knowledge are both reframed in a Foucauldian manner and extended in Gramsci-like (1971) fashion, then we could examine "the power to construct authoritative definitions of social situations" and to demonstrate how "struggles over cultural meanings and social identities are struggles for cultural hegemony" (Fraser 1989:6).[9]

Similarly, even though more materialist theories are criticized for their inability to "get at the operations of power and the possibility of resistance, . . . to comprehend the constitution and transformation of power at the level of the local and the everyday" (Martin 1988:6), they direct us to the importance of the social and historical conditions in which action and meanings, power and resistance, intellectual and expert are produced. Just as a radical feminist position can be transformed to include both a Foucauldian notion of interpretation and more structural considerations, so, too, can more materialist positions be revamped to simultaneously address both interpretive and structural analyses. In so doing they can provide "an approach capable of representing human agency, social conflict, and the construction and deconstruction of cultural meanings" (Fraser 1989:9) and social action.

In the above discussions I find it striking how contradictions are accepted at the same time that ways to bridge them are suggested. In each case, what is being called for is an analysis that treats knowledge seeking and knowledge making as situated practices. I find this viewpoint particularly useful for the discussion and analysis that follow. To understand why nurses claim the deeply gendered concept of caring as the basis for a different kind of clinical practice and a more autonomous professional status as well as to ground the situated character of knowledge production, I situate the institutions of medicine and nursing, positioning them in their historical, cultural, and structural locations.

SITUATING MEDICINE AND NURSING

The ways medicine consolidated its monopoly and professional dominance are central to an understanding of why nursing may have based its professional claims on caring. In this history adding caring to curing emerges as one of the few options available to the nursing profession—as the only game in town.

Doctors gained their professional dominance in the United States during the nineteenth century by competing in a loosely organized field of medical providers—a field not dominated by any one group.[10] At first, since there were no educational requirements, no system of formal training, and no licensing involved in claiming the title of doctor, all manner of people were free to take up the practice of medicine.

At that time no one had a clear idea about how the physical body functioned; there was no medical science or technology as the Western world understands them today. Thus there was considerable license in both diagnosis and treatment. For example, Ehrenreich and English (1973) describe the dominant belief that in women the uterus and the brain competed for energy. The use of one limited the potential use of the other. Education and the concomitant development of the brain were believed to lead to the atrophy of the uterus.[11] Since women's primary function was reproduction, upper-class women were encouraged to concentrate their physical energy on their wombs. In so doing, they would preserve their reproductive capacity while protecting themselves from the sickness, exhaustion, and injury that were routine in the lives of working-class women.[12]

Women's reproductive organs—uterus and ovaries—were characterized as controlling both body and psyche. Such characterizations led to an array of bizarre and dangerous treatments from total bed rest for the female malady of hysteria to the application of leeches to the breasts, labia (external lips of the genitals), and even the cervix (Ehrenreich and English 1973). While the medicalization of women's natural bodily processes made them more vulnerable to potentially dangerous treatments, men were not immune. In the name of medicine, the standard medical treatments for both men and women were dangerous. Both were bled and given violent purges as well as heavy doses of mercury-based drugs and opium.

In this light it is hard to contend that those who came to be called "regular" doctors gained their ascendance—their professional dominance, medical monopoly, and cultural authority—solely because of their medical knowledge and technical skills. In fact, the inadequacy of their practice, particularly the application of the kinds of "heroic therapies" just discussed, undermined the status of regular doctors and lent support to the less interventionist practices of their competition (Stevens 1966). From this perspective, the consolidation of the modern medical profession is best understood as more of a social and political victory than a scientific or technological one.

In their drive for professional monopoly, regular doctors struggled to gain control over the market for their services and over the organizational hierarchies that govern medical practice, financing, and policy (Starr 1982). At various times they lobbied for reforms, from standardizing entry into the profession and changing curricula to establishing licensing requirements. Reforms of this nature would grant them an exclusive right to practice medicine and, in so doing, transform them into an elite profession.

The elite professional status regular doctors sought was based on education and not birth; nevertheless, it ran counter to the more pluralistic practice of medicine that was prevalent at the time (Starr 1982). Not only were there many different kinds of practitioners, from bone setters to midwives and from Thomsonians to homeopathists, but dominant cultural beliefs supported individuals' right to choose the ways they wanted to practice medicine as well as the ways they wanted to be cared for. Furthermore, health care was still considered largely a family matter. Women cared for their families, called on their kin or older women reputed to have special skills, and traded advice through an oral tradition. Information was also available in almanacs and newspapers and later in guides published by physicians.

This dominant tradition supported a wide-ranging competitiveness and was both democratic and antithetical to the elitism sought by regulars. Because of the overabundance of health-care practitioners, the commitment to pluralism limited the power, prestige, and economic opportunity of any one group. This limitation was just what the regulars were fighting against. As they continued to lobby for an elite professional standing, the tension heightened; Stevens (1966) calls it a tension between elitism and democracy.

The emergence of a university medical education with some scientific substance and the formation of a coherent guild—the American Medical Association (AMA)—played a pivotal role in changing the status of regular doctors. While the first medical school opened in 1765 (at the University of Pennsylvania, then called the College of Philadelphia) and such schools had proliferated by the War of 1812, the education offered did not resemble medical education today. Two years were required for a degree. Each year lasted for three to four months, and the second year usually repeated the material of the first; the curriculum consisted of Latin and natural and experimental philosophy (Starr 1982).

Reform of medical education did not begin until about 1870. By 1890 the more advanced schools formed a national association, which set a minimum standard, including three years of training, six months a year, and laboratory work in histology, chemistry, and pathology. The medical program at Johns Hopkins became the model for this kind of education, which promoted medical training as a field of graduate study rooted in basic science and hospital medicine. The combination of high entrance requirements, a four-year curriculum, association with a major hospital, and a radically new kind of nurse-training school[13] placed Johns Hopkins in a class by itself, ahead of "any other school in the United States, in Britain, and probably in the world" (Stevens 1966:57).

While medical education for regular doctors became a field of graduate study that took as its goal a firm connection between science and research on the one hand and clinical practice on the other, the education of "irregular" doctors was taking a different path. They trained in their own medical colleges or proprietary schools. Starr (1982) calls these "commercial schools" to distinguish them from the universities, which were the domain of the regulars.

At this point, the United States was well on the way to institutionalizing two different kinds of doctors with important differences between them—the scientist/clinician and the general practitioner. The training of irregulars, those I am calling general practitioners, was quite different from the training of the scientist/clinician. It was not dependent on a university education. In addition, unlike the university medical schools, which catered to the urban, university-educated, male members of the upper classes, commercial schools had students who were more rural, more working, and lower class, and more often African Americans and women. Where regular doctors were more likely to have urban practices and treat affluent patients, the irregulars were more likely to have rural practices and to treat the less affluent.

But instead of institutionalizing two levels of health care, as many other countries did, the United States institutionalized one. In Britain, for example, the medical profession developed from three guilds—physicians, surgeons, and apothecaries. The nineteenth-century surgeon-apothecaries became the twentieth-century general practitioners, while the nineteenth-century physician-surgeons became the twentieth-century hospital-based consulting specialists. In the United States even though few university medical schools initially met the standards being set and commercial medical colleges continued to grow, the Johns Hopkins model of medical training was institutionalized and produced one kind of medical practitioner—the scientist/clinician. To reach this end, the medical profession had to become much more cohesive than it had been.

At about the same time that university schools were forming, a national organization, the AMA, was becoming a force to be reckoned with. Starr (1982) points out that for the first half of the nineteenth century, the national organization of regular doctors had few members, scant resources, and little power. It did have considerable competition within the nascent profession and a whole range of outside challenges. However, in their drive for professional and economic control, the regulars who had banded together in this organization gained considerable political clout.

According to Starr, the switch to a national organization was motivated, at least in part, by prior failures. At the local level neither educational reforms nor state licensing had been successful. In fact, licensing laws had been repealed in many states, making it increasingly clear that regular doctors could not rely on the state for protection. They needed to turn their energies inward. They also could not count on piecemeal solutions. They needed to develop a national approach. By the end of the century, broad social currents facilitated the replacement of competition with common interests, leading the way to the consolidation of a strong professional organization.

As transportation and communication improved, local isolation broke down, and national organization became both easier and more necessary.[14] In addition, Starr argues that the rise of hospitals and expanding medical specialization decreased competition as it increased the interdependence of regular doctors. They now referred to each other and, in the face of rising malpractice suits, protected each other. One benefit of the new spirit of cooperation was lower insurance costs.[15] Finally, in the name of unity and in the interest of increasing referrals, the AMA moved to accommodate some of its old adversaries, assimilating two of them—homeopathy and Electicism—into the medical profession.[16]

The consequences of this consolidation were immediate. Competition, while not eliminated, was reduced, and the AMA grew in strength. It became a large, well-financed professional organization; it published a journal and influenced public opinion. In 1904, after it was reorganized, the AMA established a Council on Medical Education and claimed education reform as its top priority. Using its ties to the newly formed foundations, Rockefeller and Carnegie, and to government bodies (Brown 1979)—ties cemented by class, race, gender, and professional interests—regular doctors now had the potential to gain the professional dominance they sought.

The gateway to economic security and professional prestige was blocked by an oversupply of health-care providers—both regular doctors and a range of irregular providers. Not only did the irregulars have large followings, but, perhaps even more important, they did not share the class and race of the regulars. The class and race positions of the irregulars diminished the image of a physician by making it more coarse and common than regulars thought was seemly. At one and the same time, then, the existence of irregular practitioners both reinforced a diminished status for regular doctors and was an economic threat. However, professional ethics forbade regular physicians from publicly opposing fellow providers, whether they were regular or irregular doctors (Starr 1982). Instead, after completing an internal report grading existing medical schools in 1904, the AMA invited the Carnegie Foundation to evaluate the admission requirements, curricula, facilities, and faculty of all medical schools then in operation.

The class, race, and gender ties between the foundations and the AMA are evident in the choice of investigator for the Carnegie Foundation evaluation: Abraham Flexner. He had attended Johns Hopkins University and taken his bachelor's degree there. His brother, Simon, held an important position in the Rockefeller Institute for Medical Research (Starr 1982). It is interesting to speculate on why the weaker medical and commercial schools gave Flexner the information he sought. Starr (1982) suggests they hoped that Flexner, as a representative of a well-endowed foundation, would provide money to bring their facilities up to an agreed-upon standard. However, he did not. Instead, he recommended that first-class university medical schools and a few from the middle ranks be strengthened on the model of Johns Hopkins; and he claimed that once they were, other schools would no longer be necessary. In fact, he suggested that only one school in each large population center was needed and that schools should admit far fewer medical students than they had been. This recommendation guided major foundations' investment in medical education (Starr 1982, Stevens 1966). For the subsequent two decades—crucial decades—foundation money went only to a select group of medical schools.[17]

The consequences of the Flexner report and of subsequent foundation funding were far-reaching. Competition among regulars and between them and the irregulars was largely eliminated. Since proprietary schools received little to no financial support, they could no longer compete, and many closed (Stevens 1966), including five of the seven schools for African Americans. In addition, only those university schools that met Flexner's criteria received financial support. As a consequence, the number of education facilities was dramatically reduced.

From shortly thereafter and thence forward, the supply of physicians did not keep pace with the population, and regular doctors, as a group, became increasingly more uniform. The high cost of a university and medical school education severely limited the number of students from low- and working-class backgrounds, while deliberate policies of discrimination against Jewish people, women, and African Americans promoted even greater homogeneity (Starr 1982). These changes contributed to increasing geographic maldistribution. While there were still practitioners to serve affluent urban communities, those who served poor and rural communities largely disappeared. At best, these communities became underserved. At worst, they often went unserved for years (Starr 1982, Stevens 1966).

While its success was not absolute, the medical profession succeeded in controlling its numbers and in eliminating most rival practitioners. The exceptions were osteopaths and chiropractors, who, after a vehement battle, were able to obtain licenses to practice; however, they were unable to win either hospital privileges or the right to prescribe drugs (Starr 1982). Overwhelmingly Americans were left with only one kind of doctor—a white, male, middle-class professional who practiced high-technology and scientific medicine with a strong emphasis on acute specialties rather than preventive primary care.

Even though the medical monopoly, professional dominance, and cultural authority of physicians may seem inevitable today, other alternatives were available. The impetus for change could have come from colleges, licensing boards, the state, or the public, rather than the AMA. Change could have been directed toward upgrading medical standards by determining the minimum qualifications necessary for protecting the public (Stevens 1966). More than one kind of doctor could have emerged. There could have been both rural and urban providers with both scientific and primary-care orientations. A few schools like Johns Hopkins could have been helped to train scientists and specialists, while many others could have been encouraged to train general practitioners to deal with common medical problems, which make up the bulk of medical practice (Starr 1982). Public needs would have been met rather than the needs of the medical profession for increased financial security and professional status.

Instead, in a struggle more social and political than scientific—a struggle with clear class, race, and gender implications—variety was removed from the practice of medicine and a self-serving version of democracy was promoted in medical education. Entry barriers to the profession were created, but once accepted into medical school all received the same basic training, with specialty training superimposed on this basic level. Since everyone received basic training, everyone was capable of being a general practitioner, and medical education was thus reconfigured as egalitarian.

Whether we agree with this reconfiguration or not, at least from the Flexner report in 1910 forward those who did not add a specialty—who remained general practitioners—occupied an untenable position. On the one hand, they were defined as specialists and their specialty included good psychological skills. These were the "specialists" charged with the task of providing comprehensive primary care for the whole family. On the other hand, they were locked in a competitive market and engaged in what proved to be an uphill struggle against an increasingly strong technological elite.

This sounds much like the position nurse practitioners find themselves in today. They are primary-care specialists with good social psychological skills, and they are locked in a battle for professional autonomy with a strong technological elite. But there are important differences. For better and worse, they are not doctors. They entered the medical field after the medical profession solidified its hold and in response to changing social conditions in the sixties.

With the passage of Medicaid and Medicare, the federal government made it economically feasible to expand the supply of physicians, which had been kept artificially low since the time of the Flexner report. The government intended to improve the availability of basic medical care, particularly in rural and inner-city areas, which physicians usually avoided (Eastaugh 1981, Morris and Smith 1977). However, from their inception, these caregivers were defined in ways that did not threaten the status, privileges, and economic security of the medical profession.

At the same time that "physician extenders" came into being, the government increased subsidized loans for medical students and financial support of medical schools (Crowley et al. 1984). From 1965 to 1982, the number of allopathic (regular) medical schools increased from 89 to 127, and the number of first-year students doubled (Tarlov 1983). But, perhaps most important, the scope of practice for physician extenders was controlled. After a hard-fought battle the official definition of nurse practitioners was changed to emphasize both their independence and their collaborative working relationship with physicians (Graduate Medical Education National Advisory Committee 1979); however, the ability of nurse practitioners to practice autonomously was severely restricted.[18]

The policies of both Medicaid and Medicare reinscribe nurse

practitioners' dependence by limiting their payment to either a health-care institution or a supervising physician. While the salaries of nurse practitioners employed by hospitals and other caregiving institutions are covered by federal reimbursement, in noninstitutional settings payment of salaries is prohibited for medical services not rendered by physicians. The only exception is for services "furnished as an incident to a physician's professional services of a kind which are commonly furnished in physicians' offices and are commonly either rendered without charge or included in the physician's bill" (quoted from a government document in Ruby 1981:768). The reimbursement practices of the insurance industry make this dependence even clearer; they pay nurse practitioners only if their services are rendered under the direct supervision of physicians. Although limiting nurse practitioners' ability to practice independently limits their ability to compete with physicians and preserves the medical monopoly over health care physicians won in the nineteenth century, it does little to mitigate the problems of the rural and inner-city people who are underserved. The Rural Health Services Act, enacted in 1977, set out in part to remedy this problem by enabling rural health clinics to receive federal payments for services provided by nurse practitioners working under the indirect supervision of and in consultation with physicians.

Given this history, the institutional forces arrayed against nursing are clear, and it is easy to understand why nursing placed caring rather than, for example, the development of a community/home-based system of primary health care or the incorporation of alternative healing practices at the center of its struggle. Even though both caring and joining physicians in a team approach to the delivery of health care have reinforced nurses' gendered identity, the gendered nature of the nursing profession, and nurses' secondary status as women and health-care providers, these options may, in fact, have been among the few opportunities nurse practitioners had for developing a clinical practice and increasing their professional status.

This history also provides ways to understand why the situated character of knowledge production may be so different in the medical and nursing professions. While both doctors and nurse practitioners have technical skills and medical knowledge that patients lack, their location in a nexus of cultural and structural factors is quite different. From its inception nursing has been subordinate to medicine, at the margins of the healing profession, and on contested terrain. While doctors were overwhelmingly male, nurses have been almost exclusively female. Where doctors were able to consolidate and homogenize their ranks by class, race, gender, and professional training, nursing has historically been much more stratified.

REDEFINING THE TERMS OF THE STRUGGLE

Since 1965, with the development of programs to train nurses in response to critical shortages of doctors, and especially since the 1975 passage of the Nurse Training Act, there has been a continuing battle over the limits of nursing and of medical practice. Today, with a growing health-care crisis, it is time to redefine the terms of this battle. To do so the claim that nurses do it better, that they add caring to curing, needs further substantiation. We need to substantiate what nurses actually do in examining rooms with detailed descriptions of their clinical practices. In other words we need information about how they nurse wounds.

By juxtaposing the ways doctors and nurse practitioners provide health care, such a study could shed light on the policy-related question about the limits of medical and nursing practice. It could also provide information related to central theoretical and methodological questions posed in this project. An in-depth analysis could provide important empirical information about how practitioners deliver health care—about caring as practice. It could also illuminate differences and similarities in the ways nurse practitioners and doctors provide care, addressing theoretical issues about the viability of caring as a discourse of the social that remedies the problems all too often associated with the medical relationship.

Information of this kind would provide the basis for a new kind of analysis and, in so doing, could be useful in nursing's struggle for professional autonomy and in current policy negotiations about how to reorganize the health-care delivery system.[19] This analysis would be both structural and interpretive. It would examine how power and resistance are produced and dismantled in situated social practices, especially as they occur in disciplinary institutions like medicine and nursing, where providers are authorized to construct authoritative definitions of social situations.

By expanding what counts as political to include the social practices through which authoritative definitions are constructed and by locating them in two different professional sites with a plurality of agents, this analysis would explore how power circulates in and through the production of multiple crosscutting discourses. It would also illuminate how these discourses promote criteria of truth and falseness as they both elevate some persons, through their institutional locations, as experts authorized to offer authoritative knowledge claims and exclude others. In addition, by analyzing the language-mediated activities of providers and patients during medical and nursing consultations and identifying both the production of discourses and conflicts between competing discourses, this analysis would clarify how these struggles over cultural meanings and social identities are also conflicts over structural and institutional interests and as such are hegemonic struggles—struggles that may be quite different in the institutions of medicine and nursing. It is to this analysis that I now turn.

THREE

COMPLAINTS MARKED AS SOCIAL PSYCHOLOGICAL
The Medical Consultation

Social science researchers, myself among them, have documented a doctor-patient relationship characterized both by an asymmetry between provider and patient (Waitzkin and Waterman 1974, Fisher 1986, Davis 1988) and by an almost exclusive concern with medical topics to the nearly total exclusion of the social/biographical context of patients' lives (Todd 1989, Mishler 1984). Nurse practitioners claim to offer an alternative, a system of care that integrates the medical and the social psychological. This system sounds much like the humanistic, patient-centered medical practices called for by reformers like Mishler who depict attention to the social psychological context of patients' lives as a remedy for the asymmetry in the provider-patient relationship. Both the arguments of reformers and the claims of nurse practitioners rest on a distinction between what Mishler refers to as the voice of medicine and the voice of the patient's lifeworld.

Against this background I chose the encounters I am about to discuss. The patients are all women, but there are important differences among them. Not all are young, working-to-middle class, and struggling with domestic responsibilities and participation in the labor force. Nor are they all old, poor, single heads of households struggling with their sexuality and their participation in heterosexual relationships. Nevertheless, in other significant respects these encounters represent the patterns I found to dominate the larger corpus of materials—patterns that I discuss in detail in the following chapters. In addition, I found that the contrasts between complaints marked as social psychological and those coded as medical

provide fertile sites at which to compare and illuminate these patterns. In Chapters Three and Four the presenting complaints are
easily marked as social psychological, while in Chapters Five and
Six they are just as easily coded as medical. Yet, the relationship
between the medical and the social psychological may be much
more complex than these distinctions indicate.

The analysis in these chapters is motivated by a series of questions. How do doctors and nurse practitioners talk with women patients whose complaints are identified as social psychological or
medical? Do the ways doctors and nurse practitioners deal with
these complaints differ? Are there two distinct voices, with providers speaking in the voice of medicine and patients speaking in the
voice of the lifeworld? Do nurse practitioners provide care that integrates the medical and the social psychological, nursing both
physical and social psychological wounds, while doctors do not? If
nurse practitioners add caring to curing, does doing so minimize
the asymmetry in the provider-patient relationship and maximize
the patient's input into the consultation?

In other words, could the inclusion of a social discourse remedy
the "troubles" in the medical encounter that Mishler and many
others have identified? Alternatively, as Silverman (1987) argues, is
this distinction between the medical and the social too simple? Can
providers and patients speak in either voice, and does a field of
power form to govern them both? Or do both Mishler's call for a
discourse of the social and Silverman's claim about the nature of
power and the ability of provider and patient to speak in a common
voice present the provider-patient relationship as if it were independent of the larger social and cultural context? Is the provider-
patient relationship, as Waitzkin (1983) posits, more accurately
characterized as deeply political?

Each of these explanations is in opposition. For Mishler the inclusion of the social/biographical context of the patient's life fixes
the medical encounter by humanizing it. But for Silverman the distinction between the social and the medical is itself problematic. He
describes these voices as interrupting each other and in this process
producing the power that governs the provider-patient relationship.
For Waitzkin neither of these explanations contains an adequate
understanding of power. They both treat the medical encounter as

if it existed in a vacuum. For him, it does not. Quite the contrary. The provider-patient relationship reflects and reinforces larger structural and cultural arrangements.

Rather than continuing these oppositional analyses, I describe the ways doctors and nurse practitioners talk to patients whose complaints are located as social psychological or medical, analyzing these descriptions by drawing on the insights of each of the theoretical positions just presented while refiguring the discussion. Instead of focusing on the either/or distinctions these theories pose, I treat the differing deliveries of health care as situated practices and locate them in specific historical, cultural, and structural arrangements. In so doing I explore how the institutions of medicine and nursing provide distinctive sites for the delivery of health care, the production of knowledge, and the negotiation of identity.

In each case, with the permission of provider and patient, I taped the consultation and transcribed the tapes for later analysis. I examine the transcripts for recurrent patterns in form—the discourse structure—and content, analyzing who speaks and how they speak, who resists and how they resist, who prevails and how they prevail. But, in addition, my attention is directed toward what is represented and how it is represented. I analyze how, as providers and patients speak in social and medical voices, their representations do ideological work and how this social/ideological work is done similarly or differently in medical and nursing encounters. In other words, in these chapters my focus is on medicine and nursing as sites at which the relationship between provider and patient, the medical and the social, medicine and society is produced, reproduced, or undermined and on how in this process gendered and professional identities are negotiated.

I chose the cases I discuss in Chapters Three and Four for their comparability. Both the doctor, Doctor Aster, and the nurse practitioner, Katherine Heinz, are primary-care providers—family medicine and community medicine, respectively. Family practice shares with nursing a commitment to patient-centered, holistic medicine, which integrates the medical and social psychological. In these cases, then, the stated intentions of both the medical and nursing practices are quite similar.

The patients, Wendy Foster and Prudence Batson, are young

women—twenty-five and twenty-seven years old, respectively. Both of them are married, are mothers, and live in intact nuclear families. While Wendy is a new mother of a first child, Prudence has three small children. They each live out a double day, working and having primary responsibility for childcare and housework. Wendy works part-time as a sales representative with her husband, and Prudence works full-time alongside her husband in a factory. Both of them are Caucasian and working-to-middle class, a fact evidenced in their ability to pay for health care.

Both doctor and nurse practitioner are meeting the patients for the first time. In each case, on this initial visit the patients have sought medical attention for vague and nonspecific complaints. Wendy's presenting complaint is that she felt faint and nauseated, and nearly passed out. Prudence's primary complaint is fatigue. Complaints of this kind, where no organic pathology is found, are often attributed to psychological rather than physiological distress.

One of the most immediately apparent differences in these doctor-patient and nurse practitioner–patient interactions is their length. The doctor-patient encounter from beginning to end provides a transcript of eight and a half pages. The nurse practitioner–patient transcript is forty pages long, and that just takes us to the physical examination. The medical consultation looks all too much like the interactions Mishler and others, myself included, have documented. It is characterized by pointed questions, a narrow focus, and a technical fix. On the surface the nurse practitioner–patient interaction looks quite different. Katherine uses open-ended questions and probes broadly for the context of the patient's symptoms.[1] Moreover, her treatment recommendations emphasize the social rather than the technical.

The medical consultation begins with Doctor Aster walking into the examining room where the patient, Wendy Foster, is sitting dressed on the examining table. She is young (twenty-five years old), Caucasian, neatly dressed, and well groomed. Her medical file identifies her as married and as having medical insurance.

    D. I'm Doctor Aster. What can I do for you today?
    P. Well, this morning I nearly passed out and my whole

body felt like it was going numb (D. Uh huh.)[2] in here; it goes through this sort of tingle. (D. Uh huh.) I just felt like that all over. Then my arms started hurting, and I couldn't open my hands, mostly my left hand but my right hand was doing a little bit but . . .[3] (D. Okay, okay.) I felt a little bit nauseated, but that's passed; but I got real feverish//[4]

D. Did this happen all of a sudden this morning or//

P. Uh hm.

D. What were you doing when it happened?

P. Feeding my baby's breakfast.

D. How old are your babies?

P. Um, six, six months.

D. Okay. More than one?

P. No.

D. Just one?

P. Just one.

There is more going on in these opening exchanges than a first glance would suggest. On the surface doctor and patient are engaged in rather routine medical talk. They greet each other, and the doctor asks how he can be helpful, providing a space for the patient to present her complaint—a medical complaint. He follows through with what appears to be routine medical questions. Yet, from the opening moment of the consultation and throughout it, social/ideological assumptions penetrate what is presumably medical discourse. As doctor and patient are exchanging routine medical information, status differentials are produced and maintained. The doctor enters the examining room clothed in the marks of his profession. He is wearing a white coat and has his stethoscope prominently displayed. He stands in front of the patient, who, although dressed in street clothes, is seated on the examining table. While the doctor introduces himself by title and last name, he does not greet the patient by name even though it is clearly marked on the file he takes with him into the examining room; and she does not object. Subtle as they are, these verbal and nonverbal communications do social/ideological work. Doctor Aster presents himself as the professional, the dominant medical expert, and Wendy as the subordinate patient; and Wendy does not resist his definition of the situation. Both in what is said and done and in what is not, dominant cultural assumptions about the identities of doctors and patients are reinscribed.

These identities can be read in the discourse. In response to the doctor's initial question, the patient tells him what happened to her that morning. She felt dizzy, had a tingling sensation in her body that felt like her whole body was going numb; her arms began to hurt; she felt nauseated, like she might pass out, and feverish. Here the doctor interrupts and asks pointed medical questions: whether the symptoms began all of a sudden and what the patient had been doing. He finds that the onset was sudden. The patient was feeding her "baby's breakfast" when the symptoms began. Then, rather than continuing to discuss the medical symptoms, the doctor switches topics and asks a rather narrowly defined social question. He asks how old the "babies" are. It seems clear that a misunderstanding is in progress. When Wendy said she was feeding her "baby's breakfast," it was unclear whether she was feeding breakfast to more than one baby or feeding one baby his breakfast. Dr. Aster seems to be assuming there is more than one baby, and though Wendy pauses and stumbles, she does not correct him. She answers his question, telling him how old the baby is: "Um, six, six months." The doctor, not the patient, clarifies. He asks whether there is more than one baby, and the patient says no. He repeats his question saying, "Just one?", and she responds in kind, "Just one."

These exchanges, too, do ideological work. The doctor, in the pursuit of a diagnosis, asks questions and initiates topics, and the patient responds without resisting, even when there is a misunderstanding she could easily set straight. The doctor, not the patient, moves to correct the misunderstanding about the number of babies. The doctor switches from a discussion of Wendy's medical symptoms to a social topic—babies. And while he seems to be asking the patient to speak about the social/biographical context of her life, on closer inspection his move from a medical topic to a social one is more ideological than inquisitive.

The doctor not only shapes the discussion but defines what is medically relevant and what is not, and he does so with little interference from the patient. The doctor never fully explores the patient's medical symptoms or moves beyond narrow and ideologically defined social topics. It is as if he has a two-place logic. Once he defines Wendy's symptoms as social psychological, he neglects her medical symptoms. Once he defines the social in narrow ideological terms, he never moves beyond this definition. Throughout the consultation he persists in seeking the cause of Wendy's symptoms in her domestic arrangements. These actions support the asymmetry of the medical relationship with its dominant medical provider and subordinate patient as they recirculate a particular version of reality that reinscribes the traditional nuclear family and women's roles in it.

This work is clearly in evidence as Doctor Aster moves to clear up the misunderstanding about the number of babies. He asks a question and receives an answer. Even though Wendy states in a clear and unambiguous fashion that there is only one baby, the doctor does not accept her response. He recycles it and checks again, "Just one?"; and she confirms again that she was feeding only one baby. These exchanges send subtle social/ideological messages. Recycling often signals a disjuncture between what is expected and what is received. While the transcript indicates how the misunderstanding about the number of babies occurred, Doctor Aster seems to have difficulty accepting that his understanding is not the correct one. Despite a clear answer from the patient, he checks again. Both recycling and checking support traditional understandings of the doctor-patient relationship. In addition, they suggest that Wendy is not a competent patient—a suggestion with a clear gender implication.

In the next exchange Doctor Aster continues exploring the social context of Wendy's life—albeit within the same narrow ideological framework.

> D. Uh, the baby's healthy?
> P. Yeah.
> D. Okay, and was anything else going on, you know, or, or just feeding the baby?
> P. No.
> D. Were you having to get your husband off to work or anything, or just . . . ?
> P. No, I'd just gotten up, and, you know (D. Uh huh.), of

course, when the baby cries, that's when you have to get up
and feed him.

    D. Was the baby upset, or was the baby eating okay, or
. . .?

    P. No, he was eating.

    D. He was eating all right?

    P. He was eating fine.

While presumably discussing medical topics, the doctor continues to explore the social context of the patient's life, a topic
he initiates, but he does so in a particular way. Rather than asking open-ended, probing questions to maximize Wendy's voice, his
questions are constraining. He questions whether the baby is
healthy, how many children she has, whether anything else is going
on like having to get her husband off to work or the baby's being
upset or not eating well. He does not ask her what is going on in her
life, what she thinks might have caused her symptoms, or how it
feels to be a new mother. Instead his focus is narrowly ideological. It
searches for explanations in Wendy's domestic responsibilities.

These questions are interesting for two reasons. First, questions
of this kind allow only a limited exchange of information. Second,
while subtle, they do social/ideological work. The doctor recycles and checks the information the patient supplies—information
about her life. He asks whether the baby was eating. After the patient responds that he was, the doctor recycles her response, checking to make sure that the baby was eating all right. Once more the
patient responds that the baby's eating is not a problem. This recycling indicates that the information Wendy is providing is somehow
at odds with the doctor's expectations, and because it is, the recycling simultaneously questions Wendy's credibility, her competence
to provide a medical history.

The ways the doctor initiates topics and asks questions thus do
ideological work. They reinstate the doctor's institutional authority,
present Wendy as less than competent, and leave the way open
for social/ideological assumptions to structure the exchange. And
structure it they do. Both the questions and the silences—the questions not asked—are saturated with meaning. They justify the traditional nuclear family, which has at its center a mother whose very

sense of herself as healthy or sick is tied to her domestic responsibilities. By implication, when babies do not eat well or when a woman is confronted with both a small child and the responsibility of getting a husband off to work, the stress may be too much for her, and so she somatizes—she makes herself unwell. While Wendy does not resist these messages, neither does she confirm Doctor Aster's assumption. Without confirmation or resistance, Doctor Aster seems unable to continue this line of questioning. He initiates a new topic and begins to take a medical history.

> D. Okay, have you had any trouble like this before?
> P. Only, well, not with the stiffness, it, but only one other time. I felt, you know, nauseated, and my muscles tightened up, and that was when I had taken diet pills; but I'm not taking anything now, and that's just, you know, that was just one time before.
> D. Just one other time?
> P. Uh huh, that was two years ago maybe.
> D. Okay, how do you feel right now? Are you . . .
> P. I feel kind of weak.
> D. Just kind of weak?
> P. I don't ache or anything.
> D. Okay, have you ever had any serious illness with your past, with your health?

Again, the doctor establishes the topic, asks all the questions and then moves on to a new topic. While at first glance these look like quite innocuous medical questions, subtle social/ideological messages are being sent. Doctor Aster starts this exchange by asking whether the patient has ever had this kind of trouble before. Wendy reads the doctor's questions as requests for medical information, and she responds by explaining that the only time she had similar experiences was when she was taking diet pills, but she is not now taking any medication. The doctor recycles her response: "Just one other time?" It is possible to claim that Doctor Aster is just asking medical questions randomly and that the ways he recycles and checks the information provided represent his personal style and nothing more. However, my experience does not support a claim of this kind. A medical interview is not a free-ranging conversation. It is constrained both by time and by the need to make a diagnosis and recommend a treatment.

From this perspective Doctor Aster's questions are an organized search for a differential diagnosis, and the responses he recycles and the information he checks are quite telling. Again, Doctor Aster is searching for the cause of Wendy's symptoms in her domestic arrangements. Here he is looking for the cause in a habituated emotional response. Has Wendy had these symptoms before?

At this point in the discussion the patient seems unaware of the doctor's social/ideological subtext. She treats each exchange as if it were a request for medical information. From this perspective, the last question is particularly threatening. Wendy comes to the clinic reporting strange and potentially frightening medical symptoms; the doctor asks some questions and then without any explanation asks whether she has ever had any serious illnesses. From her medical frame of reference, Wendy could easily assume that her symptoms signal a potentially serious illness and that is why the doctor is asking. From the transcript and the questions that follow this one, it seems clear that Doctor Aster's "Okay" and his question are a rather standard transition to a new topic. While the patient is not privy to this information, she follows the doctor's lead, providing the information he requests without questioning him or calling him to task in any way. Both the doctor's questions and the patient's responses are functioning as an ideological forum in which dominant cultural assumptions about doctors and patients, men and women, are reinstated.

The interaction continues with the doctor pursuing a fairly routine medical history; however, both doctor and patient bring social information into what is presumably a medical discussion, albeit differently. Wendy slips social/biographical information into a response to a routine medical question: While in the middle of taking a medical history, Doctor Aster switches to social/ideological questions about Wendy's domestic arrangements.

> *D.* Okay, are you taking any medicine regularly now?
> *P.* Uh huh, I was taking vitamins for breastfeeding my baby, and I'm weaning him now, so I quit taking those.

Here, the patient tacks social/biographical information about the context of her life onto the response to a routine question usually asked during a medical history. The doctor takes no special notice of this response and continues with his medical history. Toward the middle of it he asks a series of questions about the patient's domestic arrangements.

> D. Okay, what does your husband do?
> P. What does he do?
> D. Uh huh.
> P. He is a sales rep.
> D. Okay. Do you or are you working?
> P. Part-time.
> D. What kind of work do you do?
> P. I'm a sales rep too. Yeah, I work for him (laughs).
> D. Oh, okay (laughs), was there anything that was different about this morning compared to other mornings or is this a normal one?
> P. Seemed like a normal morning.
> D. Okay . . .
> P. I've had a, the last couple of days I've had a headache. I don't know if it's a tension headache or what; but, uh, you know, uh, the last couple of days I've had headaches, and I take like, you know, Tylenol, and they go away, so (D. Okay.) like that you know.
> D. Where does your head hurt?
> P. Um, sort of on both sides.
> D. Both sides?
> P. Yeah.
> D. Okay.

Both Wendy and Doctor Aster transport social information into what is presumably medical discourse. The social/biographical information that Wendy provides makes sense. Although a history is not specifically called for by the doctor's question, she explains that she is not now taking medicine but had been taking vitamins regularly. Now that she is weaning the baby, she has stopped taking vitamins.

It is hard to understand why in the middle of taking a routine medical history, Doctor Aster suddenly asks what Wendy's husband does. Wendy also seems to have difficulty understanding the question, but, once again, she does not question the relevance of the query; she just provides the information requested. However, if we assume that Doctor Aster's questions are organized by his need to make a diagnosis and recommend treatment, then the return to social topics makes sense. He is pursuing a differential diagnosis that identifies Wendy's problem as psychological, and, using the medical model as his guide, he is searching for the psychological cause of her symptoms in the domestic arrangements of her life. He has already questioned whether there are problems with the baby's eating and whether Wendy is a hypochondriac with a prior history of similar episodes. The question about what kind of work her husband does is consistent with his search for a social cause.

This search may also be embedded in the discussion of another topic. After stumbling a bit, Doctor Aster asks whether Wendy is working. She replies with no apparent trouble that she works part-time. In response to the doctor's question about the kind of work she does, she tells him that she is a sales representative too. After explaining that she works for her husband, she laughs. I read discomfort in the laugh. Wendy seems to be uncomfortable acknowledging that she works for her husband.

The doctor's next question, about whether anything had been unusual that morning, while easier to understand, seems to take him nowhere. He signals a new topic by saying "Okay," but his voice trails off as if he now does not know what topic to initiate. Wendy grabs the conversational floor his pause provides and returns the discussion to a medical topic, although one with a clear social/biographical subtext. She explains that she has had a headache for the last two days and she does not know "if it's a tension headache or what."

Wendy has enumerated a series of medical symptoms that Doctor Aster has not pursued. In addition, she has twice inserted potentially relevant medical information into a discourse largely controlled by the doctor. She tells him why she stopped taking vitamins and that she has had a headache for the last two days. Doctor Aster does not find out why she has raised these topics. He does not ask how she is feeling now that she is weaning the baby and no longer taking vitamins or what she might be tense about.

Instead of pursuing these bits of information, he asks a narrow technical-sounding question, "Where does your head hurt?" Even this question can be understood as consistent with the search for a social cause. The location of Wendy's headache could confirm its social origins as a tension headache. But it does not, and Doctor Aster is no closer to completing the task at hand: making a diagnosis.

In these exchanges the social certainly interrupts and interpenetrates the medical. Whether medical or social topics are being discussed, social/ideological assumptions are clearly embedded in the discourse. Early in the consultation, Doctor Aster abandons the search for a medical cause for Wendy's symptoms in favor of finding a social psychological cause. From that time forward, he consistently looks for the reason for Wendy's symptoms in the social context of her life. However, for him, the social is both limited to her domestic arrangements and ideologically saturated.

For Wendy the social and the medical are both more separate and more interconnected than they are for the doctor. Wendy comes to the clinic with a problem she identifies as medical. Throughout this part of their discussion she responds to Doctor Aster's questions as if they are medical questions, as if the medical and the social are separate domains. But at the same time she presents her medical symptoms as if they are intimately connected to a social/biographical subtext, which she squeezes into the doctor's search for a diagnosis. Wendy provides the medical information that she has stopped taking vitamins in a social/biographical subtext—because she is weaning the baby. Similarly, she tells the doctor that she has had a headache and provides the social/biographical subtext that it may be related to tension. However, while Doctor Aster inquires about where her head hurts, he fully investigates neither the medical complaints nor their social/biographical subtexts. We are left with no sense of what this information means in the context of Wendy's daily life or how it is connected to her presenting complaint. This presentation seems to be signaling something that has not yet been discussed.

Both in the ways Doctor Aster shapes the discussion, initiating topics and asking questions, and in the ways he limits the social to the domestic arrangements of Wendy's life, he is reinscribing the asymmetry of the medical relationship as he is recirculating hegemonic cultural assumptions about women and the nuclear family. Wendy does not contradict him overtly. Throughout the discussion Doctor Aster has retained control over the discussion, and Wendy inserts information into it. In so doing, however, she is struggling to reshape the discussion in ways that would reflect a different understanding of her situation. But she does not prevail. Doctor Aster does not pursue the information she provides, and we still have no sense of why it is important to her.

While Doctor Aster prevails interactionally, he still has not gotten the kind of information that would allow him to make a diagnosis. He continues taking a medical history, marking his transition to a new topic by saying, "Okay, all right." Again the topic here, while social, is both narrowly defined and deeply ideological.

> D. Okay, all right, what were you feeding the baby?
> P. Cereal.
> D. How does he do with that?
> P. He eats pretty good. He's a good eater.
> D. Okay. All right//

Here Doctor Aster returns to a topic he has already covered—the baby's eating. Again, Wendy says that the baby's eating is not a problem.

Once more the doctor's questions seem to have gotten him nowhere, and he begins his transition to a new topic with the now familiar transition marker, "Okay. All right." But this time Wendy interrupts him.

> P. // You think I might have some? (Laughs. D. What?)
> You think I might have some mental problems with (slight pause) the baby?

While it seems clear from the transcript that Doctor Aster is searching for a psychological cause for Wendy's symptoms, the search has been subtle. Wendy has not indicated, until this point, that she recognizes the direction of the doctor's line of inquiry. While some of his questions may have seemed strange, he is the doctor, and as a good patient she has followed his lead, providing the information he requested. And she has done so with little overt resistance. In these last questions, Wendy seems to hear a challenge to the way she has accepted her new motherhood role. She interrupts the doctor as he is in the process of another transition to ask whether he thinks she "might have some"; she laughs and then continues, "mental problems with." After a pause she continues with "the baby."

Thus, it is Wendy not Doctor Aster who makes explicit what has been implicit. She speaks aloud the social/ideological assumptions that her medical symptoms have been caused by her emotions and that her emotions are entangled with her domestic responsibilities, especially childcare. In so doing she challenges the doctor's definition of the situation. Doctor Aster neither responds to her challenge nor answers her question. He does not tell her whether he has been implying that her symptoms have been caused by some mental problems she is having with the baby.

However this naming of the social/ideological as the cause of her symptoms allows him to make a diagnosis, which he does with apparent relief. His diagnosis firmly identifies Wendy's presenting complaint as psychological and reinscribes hegemonic understandings about women.

> D. Well, I'll just tell you what I'm thinking right now, uh, what you're describing sounds like a classic hyperventilation syndrome, which is, usually happens when you're upset about something and you cannot be aware of it, but you're breathing too fast; and when you do that, you blow off too much carbon dioxide and that makes you feel weak, makes your hands tingle, feel numb, and can make you feel dizzy (P. Uh huh.); uh, but like I say it can happen really without being aware of it or really without being upset, but I just wanted to find out if that was anything you were upset about, you know, if something was (P. Not.) going on.

The patient reads this diagnosis as a request for information and responds by filling in from the social/biographical context of her life.

P. Not really this morning; it's just that, well, like the last couple of weeks my husband's been out of town opening a new store, so I had to fill in more hours (D. More hours.); and, I think, that's what I thought my headaches were from (laughs; D. laughs.) because I had so much to do. But this morning I felt nauseated, but I just, it was just like dry heaves you know. (D. Uh huh, uh huh.) I never really did get sick, so my husband told me to put your head between your legs and breathe slower and I felt better.

D. That's a good thing to do (P. But . . .); that's a real good thing to do.

P. But then when my hands started getting numb, it scared me (D. Yeah, yeah.), so he said, "Well you better go in."

These are particularly interesting exchanges. Wendy has been explicit and challenged the social/ideological assumption that her symptoms are the result of emotional problems associated with the recent birth of her son. In response, Doctor Aster makes a medical diagnosis of "hyperventilation syndrome" and locates the cause of that syndrome in Wendy's emotions. He reveals that when people are upset about something, they breathe too fast and blow off too much carbon dioxide. Doing so causes the symptoms Wendy described, and they hyperventilate. Since his questions have not uncovered a social cause, he defends his diagnosis—and by association justifies his line of inquiry—by saying that this chain of events can be set in motion without the person's being aware that she is upset. Nevertheless, he wanted to find out whether anything was upsetting Wendy. Wendy reads both his explanation and his justification as a request for information, and she provides it from the social/biographical context of her life. She explains that while she was not particularly upset that morning, she has been under some stress for the last couple of weeks. Her husband has been out of town opening a new store, and she has had to fill in more hours. She laughs as if to indicate her discomfort with the explanation she is providing and concludes that the stress of her husband's being away and the extra burden of work may have produced her tension headaches.

Even though Doctor Aster has not addressed the full range of Wendy's presenting complaint, she does not seem to take exception to the diagnosis of hyperventilation. In addition, she and Doctor Aster seem to agree that the cause for her symptoms resides in the social/biographical context of her life. However, their agreement ends here. From this point on the struggle over what are essentially contradictory definitions of Wendy's life emerges much more clearly. This struggle makes competing discourses about women and motherhood, doctors and patients, and men and women explicit for the first time. For Doctor Aster, Wendy's domestic arrangements produce an emotional conflict that causes her to hyperventilate. While Wendy does not specifically address hyperventilation, for her, specific conditions increased her work load and added an additional stress factor. These conditions gave rise to a situationally specific emotional state of increased stress. And this stress may be related to a concrete physical symptom, tension headaches.

These explanations carry conflicting ideological assumptions. Doctor Aster's explanation supports a culturally hegemonic view of women as ruled by their emotions. In addition, since he repeatedly locates the source of Wendy's emotional upset in her domestic arrangements, he also recirculates a view of women as defined by their domestic life. Furthermore, his presentation blames Wendy for her medical problems. If she could control her emotions, she would not hyperventilate. Speaking in the voice of medicine, he defines the problem as clearly social. This definition is also both ideological and political.

Wendy also defines the problems as social, and her definition is no less ideological or political. However, it provides an alternative to the dominant view of women as ruled by their emotions and defined by their domestic relationship. In addition, by resisting Doctor Aster's definition of the situation, Wendy provides an alternative to the asymmetry of the medical relationship. She represents herself as competent to define the social conditions that may have set the stage for her medical problem. As doctor and patient struggle over these different definitions, they are simultaneously struggling over culturally contradictory versions of the doctor's professional status and the patient's gendered identity. But try as she does, Wendy's definitions do not prevail.

In addition, a diagnosis of tension or hyperventilation does not tell the whole story for Wendy. She continues by raising a medical topic she has brought up before. She says: "But this morning I felt nauseated." We still do not know what the nausea means to her. We do know that she has mentioned it twice, once in her presenting complaint and again now; she expands this complaint by saying that she had the dry heaves. Wendy has now slipped four pieces of information into the discussion—nausea and the dry heaves, recent headaches and tension, the fact that she is no longer taking vitamins because she is weaning the baby, and the fact that for the last couple of weeks her husband has been out of town and her work load and stress have increased.

The doctor pursues none of this information. Moreover, even though he claims that he wants to find out whether anything is upsetting Wendy, whether something is going on in her life, the doctor neither asks the kinds of questions that might provide social/biographical information of this kind nor pursues the hints Wendy provides. Rather than exploring Wendy's nausea, a medical topic, or her tension, a social topic, Doctor Aster comments on the recommendation her husband gave her to put her head between her legs and breath slower. He says, "That's a good thing to do . . . a real good thing to do."

One of the consequences of Doctor Aster's line of inquiry is that he does not have a complete picture of the patient's medical complaints or of her life. Another is that by locating the problem in her domestic arrangements he settles for a gendered explanation and reinstates a hegemonic view of women, men, and the family. In so doing he presents both husbands and doctors as having definitional authority. And there is an additional consequence. If Wendy's symptoms are emotional not medical, perhaps the decision to come to the doctor was not a competent one. Wendy seems to hear this message, and she responds by borrowing some authority from her husband. She justifies her behavior, explaining that she got frightened when her hands started to get numb and her husband suggested that she go to the doctor. Here, the patient participates in reproducing the traditional nuclear family with a father/husband who knows best.

With the diagnosis said aloud, Doctor Aster does a brief physical examination, and, not finding anything to contradict his diagnosis, he returns to and reinforces it.

D. Okay (pause), okay, after you put your head down between your legs and, you know, started breathing slow, how long was it until you started feeling better?

P. Oh, just maybe a minute. (D. A minute.) A few seconds, really.

D. Uh huh, okay. Well, I really feel, you know, pretty strongly that that's what you were having, you know, was the hyperventilation syndrome; uh, what you did was a good thing to do, what your husband told you to do. Another thing that you could do, if that doesn't work, is to get a paper bag and make a real tight seal around your mouth and just breathe into that and, you know, attempt to build up the carbon dioxide in your blood. Uh, now, the reason as to why you had it, you know, it sounds like you are under more stress than you are normally used to. Um, is your husband going to be in town more, or is he still going to be traveling and you're gonna have to work?

P. Well, he'll be in town more now. (D. Okay.) The store's open (D. Oh.), but he does go out every week and with the same company.

D. Well, you know, if this continues to be a problem, you know, if you have any more episodes, then you know you might need to look into ways that you could limit the amounts of any work that you have to do; uh and I think that that would be a good place to start.

Again, without addressing her medical symptom, a symptom she has brought up more than once—nausea—Doctor Aster assures her that she did the right thing in following her husband's directions. He then checks to see how long it took her to recover from feeling dizzy. He goes on to explain other ways she could handle her hyperventilation.

Several things interest me here. First, by validating Wendy for following her husband's directions and by providing an additional set of directions for handling her hyperventilation, he is reinscribing a hegemonic view of men and women. Men, whether husbands or doctors, have level heads, while women, like Wendy, are swept away by their emotions. Second, even though Doctor Aster locates Wendy's presenting complaint in her domestic arrangements, he

medicalizes it. He does not accept Wendy's social/biographical definition of the situation—a definition in which hyperventilation is a
distinctive response to a specific set of conditions. Instead, he presents his diagnosis as Wendy's generalized, physiological response
to stress. This production is not at all consistent with what Wendy
has described. If she hyperventilated that morning, she did so as
a distinctive response to a situationally specific set of conditions.
Wendy has assiduously avoided the insinuation that this kind of
response is habitual.

If hyperventilation is a medical response to a conflict between
Wendy's domestic responsibilities and her labor-force participation,
then the medical task is to identify and then contain or control this
cause, this specific etiology, which Doctor Aster does. Wendy has
tentatively linked the stress of her husband's being away more than
usual and the extra burden of work that produces for her to provide
a context for explaining her increased tension and her recent headaches. These tentative links are transformed by Doctor Aster.
Wendy's work becomes the problem, and it explains more than her
tension headaches. It causes her tension and underlies her tendency
to somatize. With the underlying cause established and the diagnosis made, Doctor Aster is able to recommend treatment. He does
so by explaining that if "this" continues, and the "this" implied is
the tension that makes Wendy sick, she "could limit the amounts of
any work" that she does and, thus, the tension that makes her sick.

This diagnosis and recommendation for treatment do social/
ideological work. They take a psychological state, tension, and
transform it into a physiological one. They take a social issue, the
conflict between domestic responsibilities and participation in the
labor force, and transform it into both an individual problem and a
specific medical etiology. And they take a specific, contextual explanation and transform it into a generalized medical problem. Doctor
Aster builds upon Wendy's tentative acknowledgement that her
headache might be linked to the tension associated with the extra
burden of work caused by her husband's recent business pressures.
He moves from extra work, tension, and headaches to an essential
conflict between work and domestic responsibilities—a conflict that
generates tension and makes Wendy sick. These transformations
are performed even though Wendy has resisted and she and Doctor
Aster have struggled over this definition of the situation. Doctor

Aster's definition prevails, and while it does so without determining the meaning of work in this patient's life, it puts in the foreground one version of the medical relationship—an asymmetrical one— one version of domestic life—the traditional one—and one version of woman—the not-quite-competent, out-of-control, and overly emotional one—and thereby recirculates and reinscribes these meanings.

The doctor continues looking for other domestic factors that may be contributing to the patient's tension.

> D. Are you and your husband getting along fairly well?
> P. Yeah, fine. Well, see, there is the problem that I'm still getting up with the baby (D. Huh.) at night, you know, and that wears me out, so I didn't realize (D. Yeah.); I thought I was pregnant again. (Laughs; D. laughs.) Oh, no.

Wendy responds by assuring him that she and her husband are getting along just fine and then she tacks on additional social/biographical information. She is still getting up with the baby, she is worn out, and she thinks she might be pregnant again. Now the medical information Wendy has slipped into the discussion makes more sense. The encounter has been littered with clues. Her initial complaint includes nausea. She tells the doctor that she is weaning the baby and that she has been tense. She brings the topic of nausea up again and expands it to include the dry heaves. While each clue contributes to a consistent story, none is followed up by the doctor. She then makes explicit what the clues have been signaling: she fears that she is pregnant again.

Just as for much of the earlier part of the discussion Doctor Aster's social/ideological assumptions remained implicit, so, too, has Wendy's medical concern. Doctor Aster was searching for the cause of Wendy's symptoms in her domestic arrangements and doing so without making his search explicit. Comparably, it now seems quite clear that throughout much of this encounter Wendy has been trying to raise her fear that she is pregnant and has been doing so implicitly by dropping little hints. As Wendy earlier makes explicit what Doctor Aster has left implicit, she now does the same thing for herself.

At first glance Wendy's actions seem to contradict the asymmetry so characteristic of the medical encounter. In these exchanges she seems to be active, rather than passive, and interactionally equal, rather than subordinate. However, that symmetry pales when the consequences of her actions are considered. Once again the doctor's definition of the situation prevails. Just as Doctor Aster does not address whether he thinks Wendy has mental problems with the baby, he downplays her fear that she is pregnant instead of exploring why she is afraid.

> D. Well (pause), well, I'll tell you that it is a possibility, and I think it's remote . . . (unintelligible) breastfeeding; but since you are here we might as well go ahead and check it if it's okay with you. (P. Yeah.) You know, just to be safe.
> P. (Pauses for several seconds.) Okay.
> D. So I'll have a nurse come in in just a second, but, uh, if you're gonna be stopping your breastfeeding now, you do need, you know, to think about some method of contraception.
> P. When, uh, after I completely finish breastfeeding? When should I start with it? He told me before that if I took the pill, it might dry me up, but I can't take it until I start, right?
> D. Right. You need to start, uh, probably some time within the next two weeks or three weeks. I think you would.
> P. Okay. I don't know now, I just, I've got like one more feeding and that's when he wakes up in the middle of the night. (D. Uh, huh.) I feed him then, but all during the day he's on the bottle now so . . . (long pause).
> D. Okay. Well, I'd say that, uh, you know, if these problems continue to be a problem and, you know, the things we talked about don't work, then you come on back, and I'll be glad to, you know, go over it with you some more and talk to you about it. Or if there is anything you just want to see me about.
> P. Okay.

By downplaying Wendy's fear that she is pregnant, Doctor Aster circulates a common misperception. He tells her that while a pregnancy is possible, it is only a remote possibility since she is still breastfeeding her baby. Nevertheless, because she is worried and is in the office, they might as well go ahead and do a pregnancy test "just to be safe."

This is an interesting presentation on several counts. First, medically it is just plain wrong. A nursing mother can become pregnant. Second, neither Wendy's concern that she is pregnant nor the pregnancy test is treated as legitimate. Doctor Aster seems, instead, to assume that Wendy is being overly emotional. He agrees to do a pregnancy test not because he thinks one is medically necessary but on grounds that are at least partially social and ideological—to be safe and to reassure an overly emotional woman. Finally, in a struggle over competing definitions, this presentation recirculates messages about Wendy's competence as a woman and patient and the doctor's institutional authority to define what is, and is not, legitimate. These messages not only have clear gender and status implications but tip the struggle in the doctor's favor. Once again his definition of the situation prevails.

Doctor Aster continues by deferring the discussion of an important medical topic. He advises Wendy that after she stops breastfeeding she can come back and talk about birth control with him. He tells her, "If you're gonna be stopping your breastfeeding now, you do need, you know, to think about some method of contraception." Wendy then takes the conversational floor to ask medical questions. "When, uh, after I completely finish breastfeeding? When should I start with it?" It is unusual for patients to ask questions in this way. The medical interview is overwhelmingly characterized by what Mishler (1984) refers to as the voice of medicine. Speaking in this voice, doctors initiate most of the topics, ask most of the questions, and control the form and context of medical consultations. It is tempting to conclude that Wendy's ability to ask questions contradicts the characteristic asymmetry of the doctor-patient relationship—a temptation that diminishes as this exchange unfolds. Instead, we see the patient struggling to gain information she needs from the doctor and being only minimally successful.

Not only is the information provided here dubious at best, but it also sends strong ideological messages. Running throughout this exchange is the not-so-subtle message that doctors know best. Wendy's doctor (I suspect her obstetrician) told her that she could not take the birth-control pill without risking her ability to continue nursing her baby, and Doctor Aster agrees. He neither asks Wendy whether this presents problems for her nor hears her when she tries to explain that she is only nursing the baby once a day and hints that she is afraid that she will get pregnant. Instead, he supports a two-place logic—either the pill or breast milk—a logic that marginalizes Wendy's fear about being pregnant now or becoming pregnant as she weans the baby. In so doing he circulates a hegemonic assumption about women. They are, or should be, selflessly putting the needs and well-being of others, especially dependent others, above their own.

In addition, he provides no information about other birth-control options that would not juxtapose contraception and nursing. Instead, he treats the birth-control pill as the only way to control fertility. While Wendy might not have been a candidate for all the available methods, she certainly had options that were not discussed. This presentation is all too common. The birth-control pill is the most frequently prescribed method of contraception. Its prescription rests on and maintains the twin assumptions that contraception is a woman's responsibility and that most women are not sufficiently competent to use other, less-invasive methods reliably (compare Fisher and Todd 1986).

Moreover, there is a striking contrast here. Earlier in the consultation, when Wendy stated aloud what Doctor Aster left implicit—that her symptoms were the result of emotional problems—this social/ideological definition of the situation became the legitimate basis for his diagnosis and treatment recommendation: working produces stress, which causes Wendy to hyperventilate, and the recommended treatment is to stop working if the symptoms return. However, later, when Wendy finally states that she is afraid that she is pregnant and anxious about contraception, this medically related fear and anxiety drawn from the social/biographical context of her life does not change either the diagnosis or the treatment recommendation. Certainly these fears, rather than a conflict between work and domestic roles, could account for her tension, her headaches, and the way she hyperventilated that morning. A more medically relevant diagnosis, then, would be reasonable fear and anxiety produced by inadequate medical information. The treatment would be a pregnancy test and adequate contraception, not a recommendation to handle her tension better or to stop working. But while Wendy receives a pregnancy test, she receives no information about contraception, and the earlier diagnosis and treatment stay firmly in place. Doctor Aster concludes by reinforcing his social/ideological definition of the situation. He tells Wendy that if her problems continue—her somatic response to stress induced by working—and if discontinuing her work does not help, she can come back and talk about it some more. The "it" here is her out-of-control emotions.

Clearly, neither the assertive way Wendy has raised topics nor the inclusion of social talk in the medical encounter has erased hegemonic assumptions about women or the characteristic asymmetry of the medical relationship. Quite the contrary. While Wendy has provided important medically relevant information drawn from the social/biographical context of her life, the doctor's more social/ideological definition of the situation has prevailed, and the consequences are medical as well as ideological and political. Wendy has received neither adequate medical information nor good health care. In addition, while doctor and patient have struggled over competing definitions of women, work, and the nuclear family, both an asymmetrical medical relationship and dominant cultural assumptions have been reproduced.

Doctor Aster moves toward closing the encounter. He asks, "Do you have any questions?" Wendy's response continues the struggle over the conflicting social/ideological definition of the situation.

> P. No, I just didn't realize that that could do to you, a little bit of stress (D. Yeah); it just seemed like a little bit to me (D. Uh huh.) but . . .

The doctor interrupts her to correct her mistaken impression that she is under just a little bit of stress. In his response here the ideological messages are strongest.

> D. //Well, actually it may seem like a little bit to you, but to most people I think it'd be a great deal really, being a

mother, you know, and a six-month-old and working, too, and, you know, breastfeeding. All those are really, that's, those are lots of demands on your body, really. So I'd really try to think about ways that you could try to reduce that.

There is no mention of either Wendy's fear that she is pregnant or her concerns about contraception—medical information that could have changed the diagnosis and treatment recommendation. Instead, Doctor Aster sums up as if this medical information has not been provided. Even though Wendy's definition of the situation has not prevailed, she does not give up. She continues to resist the doctor's social/ideological definition and, in the process, to resist the asymmetry of the medical relationship and her status in it as the subordinate interactional partner and an overly emotional, less-than-competent woman and patient.

P. Well, it was, you know, it might just be because I had to work so much these past two weeks.

Wendy seems to have accepted the diagnosis. She hyperventilated. While she does not insist that the causes of her symptoms were her fear that she was pregnant and her concerns about contraception, neither does she accept Doctor Aster's definition. The struggle here is over conflicting medical and social explanations. Wendy is unwilling to accept that working caused her problem, a social/ideological explanation. And a struggle ensues in a social register. Wendy and Doctor Aster struggle over whether there is a necessary conflict between her domestic responsibilities and her work —a conflict that makes her sick—and simultaneously they struggle over the contested meaning of wife, mother, and the nuclear family. For the doctor, Wendy's stress is to be found in the conflicting demands of work and domestic roles—demands that can be eliminated if she does not work. He calls upon common understandings to support his position, saying that most people would find being the mother of a six-month-old, breastfeeding, and working stressful.

Wendy agrees that the situation produces "a little bit of stress."

While the problem for her has conflicting medical and social explanations, both are contextual and make sense only in the social/biographical context of her life. In her story the problem is neither work per se nor the conflict between being a mother, even the mother of a nursing infant, and working. Instead her presenting complaint is the result of the situationally produced increase in her isolation and responsibility as well as of the iatrogenically produced fears about contraception and about being pregnant again. Her husband has been away more than usual and responsibilities at work have increased proportionally at a time when she is unable to get an uninterrupted night's sleep and is more tired than she would usually be. She has gotten bad medical advice. Her doctor (obstetrician) told her that she needed birth control only after she stopped nursing—a recommendation reinforced in this medical consultation as well. She has a six-month-old baby whom she is weaning. She is down to one breastfeeding a day and is uncertain whether this limited breastfeeding offers contraceptive protection. She also seems unwilling to begin taking the birth-control pill if, as she has been told by her doctor, it will inhibit her ability to continue nursing the baby. She has felt nauseated. In this social/biographical context the fear that she is pregnant and the thought of another baby could produce the tension, headaches, and hyperventilation she has described.

These struggles over competing discourses have characterized the entire medical encounter. Early in the consultation Doctor Aster abandons the search for a medical cause to explain Wendy's symptoms in favor of a narrowly and ideologically defined social psychological one. He persistently searches for that cause in the domestic arrangements of her life. Once he locates work as the cause of her symptoms, he sticks to that definition despite information to the contrary. Wendy, offering a conflicting description of the situation, repeatedly resists. On some occasions the resistance is subtle; on others it is more overt. There are even times when she seems to subvert the asymmetry that characterizes the medical relationship. But in the end she does not prevail. Doctor Aster shapes the discussion. He not only initiates the topics to be discussed and asks most of the questions, but, even more important, he defines the information that counts as relevant and what does not. In so doing he recirculates the asymmetry of the medical relationship and their statuses in it as doctor and patient, man and woman, dominant and subordinate, competent and less so. He also reinscribes a particular version of reality that reinstates the traditional nuclear family and the appropriate roles for men and women in it.

FOUR

COMPLAINTS MARKED AS SOCIAL PSYCHOLOGICAL
The Nursing Consultation

In this encounter the nurse practitioner, Katherine Heinz, and the patient, Prudence Batson, are meeting each other for the first time. The encounter opens with Katherine walking into the examining room where Prudence sits in a chair waiting. The patient is young (twenty-seven years old), Caucasian, slightly overweight, neatly dressed, and well groomed. Her medical file identifies her as married and as having medical insurance. Katherine greets her and takes a seat. The encounter begins with Katherine introducing herself as a nurse practitioner. She, like Doctor Aster, wears the markers of her professional status—the white coat and stethoscope.[1] She also enacts her professional status. She initiates the topics to be discussed, asks questions, and controls the conversation.

> *N.P.* I see on the little slip that Martha [the receptionist] made out, that, uh, you're feeling tired a lot.
> *P.* Yeah, just tired.
> *N.P.* When did it start?
> *P.* Um, a few weeks ago. 'Cause I'm falling asleep early at night. Usually I can stay awake till eleven, eleven-thirty, and it doesn't bother me. And I've been falling asleep, like almost literally passing out, eight, eight-thirty, nine o'clock. And I'm sitting (unintelligible), and it's like I just run out. (Laughs.)
> *N.P.* Um hm. Has this been true every night?
> *P.* Mnn, well, it's almost every night. Just about. I get tired; I don't know, I don't know if it's the job or what?

The presenting complaint here is similar to the complaint in the medical consultation in the previous chapter. Both are easily coded as social psychological. In both consultations the providers have the interactional resources to establish the meaning of the complaint and shape the subsequent medical discussion.

In this opening sequence Katherine begins to encourage the patient to expand on her complaint and probes to get a little more information. In so doing she locates herself interactionally as the medical expert. However, she moves simultaneously to minimize the status difference between Prudence and herself, between layperson and professional, patient and medical provider. When she enters the examining room, Prudence is sitting in a chair waiting for her. Katherine, too, sits. She sits on a rolling stool, which places her lower than the patient. She moves close to the patient's chair and looks directly at her. This spatial location sends a clear message that is quite different from the message in the previous case. In the medical encounter Wendy sat on the examining table, and Doctor Aster stood looking down at her. Their spatial arrangements highlighted the asymmetry of the provider-patient relationship. The closeness of Katherine's stool, her location on it below Prudence, and the way she maintains eye contact minimize this asymmetry.

These differences are apparent in other ways as well. In the opening moments of the encounter and throughout it, the doctor consistently moved toward closure. In his search for a diagnosis, he narrowed the discussion by defining the information that was and was not relevant. In the process he abandoned a medical definition of the situation in favor of a social psychological one and then limited the social psychological to the domestic context of Wendy's life. By contrast Katherine, as we shall see, systematically avoids closure.

As the encounter continues, Katherine picks up the patient's cue —"I don't know if it's the job or what?"—just the kind of cue Doctor Aster let pass. She uses open-ended questions followed by a series of probes, and, as a result, a fuller picture of Prudence's life emerges—a picture with clear medical implications.

N.P. Tell me, go back about your job and tell me, fill me in a little bit about what your life is like now.

P. Um, well (laughs), let's see, all right. A normal day.

We'd get up about five-thirty; uh, we're out of the house by six-thirty and get the kids ready and all. Out to the sitter. Go to work at seven o'clock, um, and I build sides, upright panels; um, at 3:15 I get out of work. I go home.

N.P. How heavy is that work?

P. Oh, I don't know. It all depends. Oh, it all depends on the style. I don't know how much exactly.

N.P. Is it hard work?

P. Yeah, yeah, it's a lot.

N.P. Okay, so you get off at three-thirty?

P. Yeah. And then I go home and run around after the kids (laughs) 'til eight o'clock. You know, just normal things that I've always been doing. I don't know. I'm just tired. I don't know if I need vitamins or what.

N.P. And do you cook dinner?

P. Yeah.

N.P. By yourself?

P. Usually, (more quietly) usually . . .

N.P. And then the kids go to bed at eight o'clock?

P. Yeah, between seven-thirty and eight. They have to go to bed, or they don't get up in the morning.

N.P. And then you fall face forward on the floor.

P. Yeah, I go phttt (showing with her hand); that's it!

Prudence comes to the clinic complaining of being tired. She explains that she used to be able to stay up later, "eleven, eleven-thirty," but now she falls asleep around eight or eight-thirty and is "almost literally passing out." Katherine takes the patient's complaint seriously. She does not assume the problem is psychological or seek its cause in the patient's domestic arrangements. Instead, she asks Prudence to describe what her life is like. In response to this open-ended question Prudence describes what she calls a "normal day" and Katherine learns that her day starts at about five-thirty in the morning, that she has total responsibility for domestic arrangements—from taking the children to the baby sitter to taking care of the house—and that she also has a job outside the home that involves physically hard labor. When the patient gets home from work, she runs after the kids, cooks dinner, and puts the children to bed. When her responsibilities end, she feels tired. Although her being tired seems easy to understand, Prudence describes her day as normal and wonders whether she needs "vitamins or what."

Katherine does not pick up the medical cue—the need for vitamins. To do so would be to medicalize and individualize a social problem. In the prior encounter, I criticized the doctor for not pursuing the patient's medical symptom, nausea. Here I seem to be praising the nurse practitioner for a similar lack of attention. How can I account for this apparent discrepancy? Nausea and a need for vitamins are not equivalent. Nausea is a symptom, a clue in the search for a differential diagnosis. Vitamins are a treatment recommendation. Doctor Aster might have gotten medically important information by pursuing the meaning of Wendy's nausea. There is no similar gain in pursuing whether Prudence needs vitamins. At this point in the encounter Katherine does not have enough information to discuss their potential benefits. Instead of discussing possible treatments, she legitimizes the patient's experience, implying that anyone, after putting in a day like the patient describes, would be tired. She says, "And then you fall face forward on the floor."

Notwithstanding the legitimacy of Prudence's fatigue, something has induced her to seek medical attention now. Yet, although she has described a "normal day" and has explained that she is doing the things she has "always been doing," she also tells Katherine that these things did not tire her before. Katherine has a choice here. She can assume that Prudence's problem is emotional and that its source is her domestic arrangements, as Doctor Aster did with Wendy, or she can check further. Katherine probes with open-ended questions to find out whether anything has changed in Prudence's life.

> *N.P.* How long have you been working?
> *P.* Since September [almost a year ago].
> *N.P.* So the schedule has remained essentially unchanged?
> *P.* Oh yeah, yeah, it's been about the same since September.
> *N.P.* Is there any other adult in the house with you?
> *P.* My husband.
> *N.P.* What's his schedule like?

P. The same as mine. He works right next to me.

N.P. Oh, you work in the same place?

P. Yeah (N.P. Oh), same place. He works right next to me. He repairs all of the pianos that are brought in or shipped in from a lot of countries.

Prudence is consistent. While she has been describing a day that would make anyone tired, she was not tired before and is now. Katherine checks to see how long Prudence has been working and whether her schedule has changed. Prudence's explanation that her schedule has remained essentially unchanged since she went back to work seems to be at odds with Katherine's expectations. She recycles the information, checking again. We can almost see her switch gears here. If the fatigue Prudence describes is not caused by what she does during the day, does it result from some other aspects of her life?

Katherine begins again. She asks whether there is "any other adult in the house." In itself this is an interesting question. It assumes neither that Prudence is now married nor that she is in a heterosexual relationship. Katherine continues using open-ended questions and learns that Prudence is married and that she and her husband work in the same place. The nurse practitioner recycles this information. We can almost hear Katherine mentally putting her finger on this spot, wondering whether this working relationship plays a role in Prudence's fatigue.

Once again the way Katherine has asked questions provides important social/biographical information and offers her a choice. She can assume that either working or this particular work situation is the source of Prudence's fatigue. But she does not. Instead, drawing on the logic of the medical model, she continues her search for the potential sources of Prudence's fatigue. She says "okay," makes a transition to a new topic, and probes again using open-ended questions.

N.P. Okay. Does he help at all with the kids or dinner or any of that?

P. Sometimes. I've been screaming at him a lot lately, though. (Laughs.) I guess I'm mean sometimes. God, but I get so mad, you know. "Help me with dinner!" I'm, you know, gee, I get so mad at him sometimes. Just, he can take it upon himself just to walk out the door and walk over to the neighbors and have a grand ole time, not thinking, you know, "Do you want me to keep an eye on the kids for a minute while I go." You know, and I have to ask because I can't just walk out, and the kids'll be there alone. So . . . but I've really been getting on him about it lately. God, I get so mad.

N.P. How does he respond to that?

P. "I didn't know." (Mocking.) I get so mad at him. (Laughs.) But he just, and then for a couple of days he'll be fine. And then, "I have to go work on the lawn mower" (mocking, laughs), and all this other crap. You know?

N.P. Oh absolutely!

P. I'm just getting so mad at him, though; he's, he's not very helpful sometimes, a lot; he well, he is; but sometimes, you know, when it comes to cooking, and just being able to walk out of the house and go work on the lawn mower or the motorcycle or something. It's a lot; it's freedom to him, you know; it's, that's what I look at it as. Because he's got the freedom to just walk out the door and, you know, go talk to his friends or something. I don't have that. I've gotta stop and say (N.P. Sure.) somebody's gotta watch these kids, you know. (N.P. Sure.) I just can't leave them all free there, or you know I'll come home to a mess. (Laughs.)

N.P. That's right!

Katherine has not moved rapidly toward closure. She has not narrowly defined the information that is and is not relevant to the discussion at hand. Instead, she has treated Prudence as a competent person, patient, and woman able to talk sensibly about what is bothering her. At each opportunity she has given Prudence the opportunity to talk about her life and, in so doing, to explain the meaning of her presenting complaint. As a result, a picture of Prudence's life is emerging. She works hard, putting in a double day at home and in the paid labor force. But although she and her husband work side by side in the factory, he does not work by her side in their home or with their children. Prudence describes her husband as "not very helpful sometimes" and then corrects herself and explains that he is not helpful "a lot" and she is "getting so mad at him."

Although the topic here is social/biographical, the information provided is potentially important medically. Prudence reveals that her work life has remained consistent for nearly a year, but her home life has not. She describes herself as increasingly unhappy about her husband's lack of participation at home and explains that she has "been screaming at him a lot lately." He responds by being fine for a couple of days before returning to his former behavior. She is angry that he has the freedom to walk out of the house to visit the neighbors or work on the lawn mower without worrying about who will take care of the children. She is angry that she does not have a similar freedom. Her anger at her husband easily could be related to the fatigue she describes.

Again Katherine has choices. She can cut off the discussion and make a medical diagnosis. Relying on the social/biographical information Prudence has provided, Katherine can conclude that the anger and frustration the patient describes produce depression, depression induces fatigue and can be treated medically. Alternatively, Katherine can rely on dominant cultural understandings—social/ideological understandings—and assume that the patient's problem lies in a conflict between her work and her domestic roles. Prudence cannot handle the stress this conflict produces and so she makes herself sick. Katherine can then treat Prudence's complaint as a social problem. She can recommend, as Doctor Aster did, that Prudence stop working. If she did not work, perhaps she would not be as angry and frustrated as she claims to be, and the chain of causation from anger and frustration to depression and fatigue would be broken.

Katherine makes neither of these choices. Instead of medicating the patient or blaming her for the problems she is experiencing, she validates her anger and frustration. When Prudence describes how angry she gets when her husband abandons the children, saying that he has to go work on the lawn mower, Katherine says, "Oh absolutely!" When Prudence talks about her husband's freedom and her lack thereof, Katherine affirms her reality by saying "sure." When Prudence says, "Somebody's gotta watch these kids," Katherine again says, "Sure." And when Prudence explains that if she were to leave the children, she would just come home to a mess, Katherine supports her 100 percent. She says, "That's right!"

Here Katherine, like Doctor Aster in the previous consultation, is speaking a social/ideological discourse, but this discourse is different from and, in fact, is in opposition to the doctor's. Katherine neither positions Prudence as an overly emotional woman nor makes an early diagnosis. Instead, she sums up the information Prudence has provided, legitimates her feelings about her life, and, asking open-ended questions, probes to learn more.

> *N.P.* Has, you say you have been working since September and the schedule has been basically unchanged. (P. Yeah.) Has anything happened with your husband that's different? In other words, is he, is something different about the interaction in the last month or two?
>
> *P.* Um, we're not, I don't know. It's just like a, it's like two magnets. We're just, I can't seem to get close to him in the last few weeks. I just want to stay away. Maybe that's why I'm falling asleep so early. (Laughs.) So I don't have to listen to him or anything. But he gets so mad at me. Like at night, sometimes I just want to sit there and read a book or something, and he gets so mad . . .
>
> *N.P.* What's his anger?
>
> *P.* He thinks his sex life is crazy. He thinks, "Why do you want to read books, when you know it's . . . "
>
> *N.P.* When you could be having sex.
>
> *P.* Yeah, and it's not that I don't want to. I just don't want him to talk to me like that. You know? (Laughs.) And I try to tell him, but he won't listen to me. Anyway I get so mad at him.

Katherine asks what's different with Prudence's husband now, and in response the patient begins to diagnose herself. She describes herself as "just wanting to stay away" from her husband in the last few weeks and concludes, "Maybe that's why I'm falling asleep so early. So I don't have to listen to him or anything." She continues by providing additional information. "Sometimes I just want to sit there and read a book or something, and he gets so mad." Again Katherine probes, "What's his anger?" Prudence responds, "He thinks his sex life is crazy." She continues by explaining that her husband does not understand why she wants to read when she could be doing other things. Her voice trails off and Katherine finishes her sentence, "When you could be having sex." Although sex may be a problem between husband and wife, talking about it seems to pose no trouble for nurse practitioner and patient. Prudence continues by acknowledging that sex is a problem and clarifying that it is not that she does not want to but she does not like the way he has been talking to her. When she tries to tell him, he does not listen, and she gets even angrier.

The picture gets clearer here. Both husband and wife are angry —an anger that is being argued out over sex and is perhaps being acted out in Prudence's fatigue. This is not a picture imposed by the nurse practitioner. Quite the contrary. Until now she has done little more than ask questions and speak an oppositional discourse that supports Prudence's feelings. In this context, Prudence raises her husband's anger as a topic of discussion. When Katherine probes to find out more about it, Prudence links her husband's anger to sex. Moreover, it is Prudence, not the nurse practitioner, who makes the diagnosis, who names her emotions as the potential cause of her fatigue.

In my experience this is an unusual exchange. Medical providers, not patients, are usually interactionally dominant. They initiate topics for discussion. They make diagnoses and recommend treatment. In so doing they reproduce their medical authority and the asymmetry of the provider-patient relationship. In this exchange, while the patient does not initiate all the topics for discussion, she initiates some, and she, not Katherine, diagnoses her problem. It is tempting to conclude that provider and patient have changed roles, to think that the social/ideological work that produces and maintains the provider's dominance and the patient's subordinance is totally lacking. But it would be a mistake to assume that Katherine has lost control or that Prudence is now in control of the interaction.

Katherine, like Doctor Aster, reenacts the asymmetry of the provider-patient relationship. But she does so differently, more subtly, and not at the cost of the patient's competence. By initiating topics, asking open-ended questions, probing for additional information, and legitimating Prudence's feelings, she provides the space for Prudence to display her competence and even to diagnosis herself. This diagnosis maximizes the patient's input into the medical discussion, minimizes the asymmetry of the provider-patient relationship, and locates her as a competent woman and patient. But it does not challenge the provider's medical competence, her institutionally based authority. After all, this is a medical setting, and it is the provider who makes it possible for the patient to describe the social/biographical context of her life and to diagnose herself.

In this case and in the previous one, the diagnosis is quite similar. Both Katherine and Doctor Aster identify emotions as the source of the problem. But there are significant differences. Doctor Aster imposed his diagnosis. Early in the encounter he narrowed the discussion, locating the source of Wendy's problems in her emotions. Working in the paid labor force and domestic responsibilities are too much for her so she somatizes. Katherine, by contrast, does not prematurely narrow the discussion or impose a diagnosis. Instead she encourages Prudence to talk about her life and, in so doing, provides the space for her to make her own diagnosis. Perhaps even more important, she does not represent Prudence's emotions as out of control and making her sick. At every opportunity Katherine defends the patient's responses to her life. She consistently supports the view that Prudence is legitimately upset.

While both Doctor Aster and Katherine speak in a social/ideological voice, the messages they send are diametrically opposed. Where Doctor Aster recirculated dominant cultural assumptions about women, men, and relationships, Katherine does not. She consistently supports Prudence's more oppositional leanings and speaks in ways that undermine dominant cultural understandings.

Once again Katherine picks up topics that Prudence has raised—anger and sex—and probes further.

> *N.P.* Tell me about the, the difference between you over sex. How long has that been going on?
>
> *P.* Just the last few weeks. Probably since I've been going to bed so early. I don't know. Maybe it's like I'm trying to ignore the issue. You know (quietly)?

Katherine continues to probe, trying to determine when the problem with sex began, and Prudence vacillates between admitting there is a problem and claiming that she does not know what the problem is. Sex just got old about a month ago, at about the time she began to go to bed early.

Katherine certainly now has the grounds to narrow the discussion to the patient's anger, to focus in on it as the source of Prudence's fatigue, but she does not. Instead, she continues to ask open ended questions and to search for how in the last month the link between anger, sex, and fatigue was forged.

N.P. Has this happened before in your relationship?

P. Yeah. It did once before, and it was a good month or so before I, I just wanted my freedom, you know. I wanted to be able to go out and do something, not with other men or anything, you know, with my friends. Go out and have a drink with them, or just go over and visit them. I mean without him always being there. I just feel suffocated sometimes.

N.P. Un hm, I would think working next to him . . .

P. It's suffocating, and I've been sitting on this other job, on the jobs out of my department, just to get away from him. And I'd, I don't know maybe that's something psychological telling me to "get outa there," away from him. I'm next to him all day. And he's right there. It's, I feel like I'm being watched or something, you know? N.P. Does he comment on your work at all?

P. Sometimes.

N.P. What's the nature of his comments?

P. Oh, it's never, well, it's not really bad, but it's not good either. It's mostly negative.

N.P. How does he evaluate the work you do around the house?

P. He thinks I, that, I don't know. He, um. (Sighs.) The house can never be clean enough, and he makes me feel guilty if I'm outside with the kids, pushing them on the swing, when there's a floor to be swept or something. He just, "Oh the floor is so dirty and you're out there fooling around." You know, I get so mad at him. Huh! Even to talk about it even gets me angry.

N.P. I can certainly understand that.

P. Yeah?

N.P. I can tell you that I and most of the women I know would not survive in that kind of atmosphere.

P. You know, I don't want sex; I don't want nothing else to do with him until he straightens, you know, just leave me alone, for, you know, let me have a little bit of freedom, you know, some. My mother's even told him about it because he's very suffocating. Very, um, he doesn't like me to have other friends because it's, um, he's afraid my friends will, um, I don't know if it's take me away from him or give me ideas in my head. I told him, like I told him, nobody can put ideas in my head, you know, unless I want them there. . . . I want to go shopping with my friends, you know. I can have girl friends, you know. But even when we were in school, it was like that. I had a hard time keeping friends cause he was just, he's obnoxious. He's obnoxious to my family . . . I love him but he is just a jerk sometimes, you know.

This open-ended exploration produces results. Katherine learns that Prudence is angry about the inequities of her double responsibilities at home and at work. She is frustrated by the lack of symmetry in the relationship between herself and her husband. She resents her husband's freedom to walk away from domestic responsibilities and her lack of such freedom. Prudence wants to be able "to go out and do something, not with other men or anything, you know, with my friends." She feels suffocated being with her husband twenty-four hours a day. She is trying to change jobs so that she will not have to work next to him. She resents her husband's evaluations at work and at home, evaluations that consistently devalue her performance and contribute to her mounting anger. Although she says she loves him, she does not want to have sexual relations with him. She explains, "I don't want nothing else to do with him until he straightens. . . . Just leave me alone. . . . Let me have a little bit of freedom, you know, some."

By not prematurely narrowing the topics for discussion, Katherine learns that the conditions surrounding Prudence's fatigue are much more complicated than they seemed at first. The picture that emerges here presents both husband and wife as engaged in a continuing struggle over the conflicting meanings of being wife/mother and husband/father in an economic climate that makes it increasingly necessary for both husband and wife to be wage earners. While the economic context has changed, cultural assumptions that make domestic duties a shared responsibility are much slower to develop. Prudence has moved into her husband's workplace. She is angry because he resists moving into the domestic arena traditionally seen as her workplace.

While her husband's voice is not present here, it is not too difficult to read between the lines. Prudence is angry about the lack of equity in her marriage, and her husband's anger is probably triggered by her demand for equity. He is angry about the changes that have moved his wife into his workplace. He is angered by her demand that he contribute at home. And, in addition, he is angered by her increasing demand for "freedom." If he has the freedom to be with his friends and do the things he enjoys, she wants the freedom to be with her friends and do things that she enjoys. This anger gets acted out in their sexual relationship.

As this story unfolds, Katherine does not just passively receive it. She both elicits social/biographical information about Prudence's life and responds to it. In so doing she is not a neutral, objective provider, but neither was Doctor Aster. The difference is that while Doctor Aster consistently reinscribed traditional values about women, work, and the nuclear family, Katherine does not. She does not tell Prudence that her symptoms are caused by a conflict between her domestic responsibilities and her labor-force participation. She does not even imply that her stress would be reduced if she stopped working and stayed at home. Neither does she invalidate Prudence's anger or explain why it is that her husband may be angry. She does not excuse his behavior by telling Prudence how hard the changes in their lives must be for him.

Instead of reproducing a hegemonic understanding about the nuclear family and Prudence's role in it, Katherine supports Prudence and, in so doing, speaks an oppositional discourse. She tells her that she can "certainly understand" how angry she is. By supporting her anger, Katherine also legitimates Prudence's participation in the labor force as well as her desire for more freedom. When Prudence questions her support by saying "Yeah?", Katherine calls on an absent community of women to make her position more emphatic. "I can tell you that I and most of the women I know would not survive in that kind of atmosphere."

This way of gathering information and responding to it sends different social/ideological messages about provider and patient. While Katherine reproduces her professional status, this status is not built on the foundation of the patient's incompetence. Prudence is treated as the expert on her own life. Moreover, Katherine contributes to a renegotiation of their identities. While they remain provider and patient, they also relate to each other as women. By positioning herself in a community of women, Katherine identifies herself as like Prudence. On the basis of this gender solidarity she legitimizes Prudence's experiences and, in so doing, resists dominant cultural assumptions about men, women, and relationships.

Katherine is also able to obtain a much richer narrative. Where in the medical encounter Wendy had to squeeze social/biographical information into a more technically oriented discourse, Prudence is encouraged to construct and comment on the social context of her life and in so doing to give meaning to her presenting complaint. The picture that emerges of the patient's life and its relationship to her presenting complaint is not easily reduced to out-of-control emotions. It depicts a struggle between husband and wife that, while centered in the patient's sexual responsiveness, is much more far reaching.

At this point in the encounter Katherine begins to ask deeply probing questions and more explicitly to support an oppositional discourse. In so doing she sets the stage for a struggle over conflicting social/ideological discourses.

> N.P. Did you ever think of leaving him?
> P. Yeah, I thought of it a couple of times. But I don't know, it just gets so . . . I don't know, I want to stay, but . . . you know, I mean we got married when I was fifteen, you know, and it's like I never had other boy friends. I never . . . I don't know. I've always been a mother, a wife, and a

housecleaner. I want to do something else. (Laughs.) You know?

N.P. You know that's absolutely understandable. That's, that doesn't (P. Good; laughs.) make you a bad person.

P. Good (laughs), that's one reason I went out and got a job in September 'cause I couldn't handle it, being home all the time, you know, I was, just no adult conversation . . .

N.P. You know that's a real growth step for you, to realize those needs and then to go take some action, to do something about them. Do you see that as a growth step?

P. Yeah, yeah.

N.P. You do?

P. I, um (laughs), I've been keeping it so pent up.

N.P. Well, I think part of us thinks that in a way you're being a bad mother. I mean after all if you were a good mother, you'd love to sit around and be happy to play with your children. But you and I both know that is crazy. (P. laughs.) That's what we were raised to think. Good mothers would rather do nothing more than cook and clean and sweep the floor, watch the children, and hope their husbands will let them do something else for them. Right?

P. Yeah. I mean, that's what even my mother said, you know, when I first got married.

Where Doctor Aster suggested that Wendy stop working and instead concentrate on her domestic responsibilities, Katherine asks Prudence if she ever thinks of leaving her husband. This question offers an alternative to dominant cultural discourses. Rather then reinscribing the nuclear family, Katherine speaks an oppositional discourse that suggests that Prudence can leave her husband, make a life for her family, and still be a good woman. Prudence responds by saying that she has thought about leaving her husband "a couple of times." As she begins to explain, she recirculates the dominant discourse Katherine has resisted. She says, "I want to stay," and she continues by revealing why she feels as she does. "We got married when I was fifteen. . . . I never had other boy friends. . . . I've always been a mother, a wife, and a housecleaner."

But Prudence then seems to contradict herself. She says, "I want to do something else." What emerges here is a complex picture of a woman struggling with herself over conflicting discourses. She both reinscribes and resists the dominant discourses about being a wife, mother and worker. On the one hand, Prudence describes her identity in hegemonic terms. She identifies herself in relation to her domestic responsibilities. On the other hand, she wants to do something else, something other than being a mother, wife, and housecleaner.

Once again the nurse practitioner's responses are neither neutral nor objective. She supports and validates Prudence's reluctance to be contained by traditional domestic arrangements. When Prudence says she wants something more, Katherine responds, "That's absolutely understandable." She then goes on to tell Prudence that wanting to do something more does not make her a bad person. In so doing she legitimates Prudence's more oppositional desires as she names and resists the unspoken, but all too present, cultural assumption that a woman's primary responsibility is to home and family.

In response Prudence reveals that wanting more was the reason she got a job in the first place. She explains that she "couldn't handle it, being home all the time" with "no adult conversation." Prudence implies here that she is somehow failing because she cannot handle her domestic responsibilities—an implication that is easy to understand. In the dominant cultural discourses, which foreground women's domestic responsibilities, work may be an economic necessity, but it should not provide an opportunity for the pursuit of self interest, the "selfish" pursuit of individual interests. Again Katherine legitimizes her feelings by telling her that it is growthful for her to realize her needs and take steps to meet them. By encouraging Prudence to meet her needs, Katherine resists traditional domestic arrangements and, in so doing, is again speaking an oppositional discourse.

Katherine goes on to name the unspoken cultural assumptions about women that Prudence seems to be struggling with. She states aloud the dominant cultural assumption that good wives and mothers should be satisfied staying home and taking care of their husbands and children. Here again the way Katherine speaks constructs a shared sense of identity, a gendered solidarity. As she lays out the dominant cultural assumptions, she sprinkles her description with phrases that position her as a woman like Prudence—"part of *us* thinks that," "*you* and *I* both know," "*we* were raised to think"—and she ends this description by eliciting agreement. She says, "Right?", and Prudence responds, "Yeah." Here Prudence is acknowledging that she is familiar with hegemonic discourses. If the culture has not sufficiently informed her, her mother has.

This exchange makes the differences in the medical and nursing encounters quite specific. While in the nursing encounter Katherine supports an oppositional discourse and works to establish gender solidarity, she has not pressed her point of view. Prudence has struggled with herself over conflicting discourses, but at least to this point in the encounter she has not had to resist the provider's definition of the situation. When Prudence constructs her life in a hegemonic lexicon, she meets no opposition from Katherine. When she represents her life in more oppositional terms, Katherine validates her presentation.

In the medical consultation the doctor did not provide an oppositional discourse. On the contrary, Doctor Aster consistently relied on and reinscribed dominant cultural assumptions about women, men, and the nuclear family. He consistently pressed his point of view, reinforcing his professional dominance. In this process, even though Wendy struggled to get her more oppositional point of view heard and even though she resisted Doctor Aster's definition of the situation, she did not prevail. The differences in these dynamics emerge even more clearly in the discussion that follows.

Prudence has brought her mother into the conversation, and Katherine pursues the topic further.

> *N.P.* So your mother says you're not a good wife?
> *P.* Oh no, when we were first married she was like that;
> but she was married at the time, and my father left her, and
> she has changed her whole way of thinking. This woman, you
> would not believe her. I mean when she was married, my
> father wouldn't let her cut her hair. He wouldn't let her wear
> makeup. He wouldn't, you know, she was the classic
> housewife. She just, they never went out. They never did
> anything; and since she's been separated, she's changed . . . in

the way she thinks and the clothes she wears; and she has her hair done, and she's got contacts, and she tells me, "Don't make the same mistake I did."

N.P. What's the mistake?

P. Tying yourself in the house, not having any friends, not . . . I'm starting to listen to her.

N.P. You must have a bad case of the covets when you are with her.

P. I do.

N.P. So what I hear is that your father leaving your mother was good for your mother.

P. Yeah, it was. It was great. Not for the first year, but once she got over that, she just, she made a whole new turn.

N.P. So when you think about leaving your husband, do you see yourself as your mother?

P. Yeah, yeah, I'd be able to go out and have friends and do things, but . . .

N.P. What do you do with all these feelings?

P. Keep them way inside, yeah.

N.P. And fall asleep at eight o'clock.

P. And fall asleep at eight o'clock.

The picture of Prudence that surfaces in response to these open-ended questions reveals her anger and frustration. She is a woman struggling between traditional domestic arrangements and an alternative to them. Prudence feels suffocated, and going to work has not alleviated this feeling. She has gotten out of the house but has not gained any of the other freedoms she craves. Instead, she has a double day and is negatively evaluated by her husband both at home and in the factory. She has said she wants to remain married. But she also describes her mother's divorce in glowing terms and recognizes that if she divorced her husband, she, too, could have some of the freedom her mother now has. This mother, who once reinforced a traditional view of marriage and motherhood, now advises her daughter not to make the same mistakes she made, not to tie herself in the house without friends; and Prudence claims to be paying attention.

Katherine asks what Prudence does with the feelings these conflicts generate, and Prudence says, "Keep them inside." Patient and nurse practitioner then agree on the diagnosis. Keeping these feelings inside—feelings that are legitimate—produces the fatigue that sends Prudence to bed at eight o'clock each evening. The way the diagnosis is reached does social/ideological work. While the patient's input into the decision-making process is maximized, the characteristic asymmetry of the provider-patient relationship is minimized but not abandoned. In addition, by encouraging Prudence to speak about the social/biographical context of her life, Katherine makes the conflicting positions she is struggling with visible. While Prudence speaks an oppositional discourse about women, work, and the nuclear family, she also locates herself in more hegemonic terms and gives preference to them.

With the diagnosis reached, Katherine could move toward a discussion of potential treatments. But she does not. Instead, she explores whether these feelings get acted out in ways that are potentially dangerous.

> *N.P.* You know, most people, you must be very angry, beyond your ability to manage it.
>
> *P.* I am. (Laughs.) I am!
>
> *N.P.* One concern I have is that the anger is directed toward people other than your husband, like your children.
>
> *P.* Sometimes, but I don't, I've never, um, see, I was an abused child myself, so; and I don't even hit them, you know, I mean little pats, but it's like I'm afraid to because I know what it was like as a kid. And . . . they probably, I mean everyone always says, "You let the kids get away with so much." But it's my kids and I, we have a good understanding, my kids and I. We can usually, I'll say, "Get to your rooms and stay there. I'm real mad and you don't want to see me right now."
>
> *N.P.* Well, the other person that, that a lot of us take it out on is ourselves.
>
> *P.* Yeah, I'm probably in some way doing that. I go to sleep, hide away from it.
>
> *N.P.* We end up being angry with ourselves. In fact, there is a school of thought that says anger turned inward is what depression is. Do you feel depressed?
>
> *P.* Yeah. A lot. I've really changed over the last couple of

months. I've always been such a happy person. You know, I'm not anymore.

Here, Katherine returns to the social/biographical context of Prudence's life and asks two questions that are often not asked in medical encounters. Despite mounting evidence of domestic abuse, such abuse all too often goes unrecognized, unreported, and untreated. In the face of the anger and frustration that Prudence reports, Katherine asks whether she directs it toward people other than her husband, like her children. Prudence responds that she was an abused child herself. She has developed strategies to avoid abusing her children, and these strategies are successful—a response that Katherine accepts. She then inquires about depression, and, in so doing, Katherine works to produce a shared gender identity. She says, "The other person that . . . *a lot of us* take it out on is *ourselves.*" And later she continues by saying, "*We* end up being angry with *ourselves.*" Prudence acknowledges that she takes her anger out on herself and that she is depressed. With the diagnosis agreed upon and depression acknowledged, Katherine moves on to explore treatment options.

Both the topics just discussed and the following discussion of treatment options are characterized by a tension not customary in medical consultations. The nurse practitioner personifies the institutional authority associated with her professional status. At the same time, however, she works to produce and maintain a gender solidarity based in women's common experiences. Yet whether talking as a professional or talking as a woman, Katherine relies on the asymmetry that characterizes the professional-patient relationship.

Her professional status, which the patient lacks, enables Katherine to ask deeply probing questions about child abuse and depression. While these questions are undoubtedly important, they nevertheless reinscribe the asymmetry of the provider-patient relationship. Katherine's professional status and the authority accorded to it also provide the ground for her to locate herself as a woman like Prudence. In so doing she both recirculates the asymmetry of the medical relationship and distances herself from it. Here, while speaking as a woman, Katherine articulates an oppositional discourse that legitimates both the patient's experiences and her emotions. Since this is a professional consultation and not a meeting of friends, a certain tension between these discourses seems unavoidable (compare Davis 1988), and where there is tension a struggle often follows.

While a struggle has not been part of the diagnostic process, it emerges quite clearly when the consultation turns toward treatment recommendations. Katherine again returns to Prudence's life and begins to explore a variety of ways to treat the problems producing Prudence's fatigue. She starts by asking Prudence what options she sees, how she thinks she could make her life better. Prudence says that she is depressed because she cannot see any options. Katherine then returns to a prior topic.

> *N.P.* You said that you thought about leaving your husband. What has the world looked like to you when you picture yourself having left your husband?
> *P.* I want to know what I'm going to do with three kids, a car payment, the rent. You know, I . . . no way I can cut it on my own with, you know, just one salary. Forget it. There's no way.
> *N.P.* So it's economic?
> *P.* Yeah.

Katherine has raised the topic of divorce twice before and she has learned that, at best, Prudence is ambivalent—an ambivalence that sets the stage for Katherine's oppositional recommendations. Prudence is frustrated and angry about her current domestic arrangements. She sees that her mother's divorce provides some of the freedoms she craves, yet she wants to stay married. She also wants something more, a kind of freedom and equity not currently in her marriage. Here we see Prudence struggling with competing discourses. On the one hand, she presents herself as someone who can hardly imagine not being married. But at the same time she thinks about divorce. The conflict here is between being married and not being married. On the other hand, she chafes in her current marriage, with its traditional gender arrangements, and struggles to redefine it in more egalitarian terms. Here the conflict is about how her marriage is to be defined.

Katherine enters only one of these conflicts—the one between marriage and divorce—and she does so firmly on the side of divorce. She raises the topic again, and Prudence provides an economic rationale for being unable to consider a divorce. Katherine takes these economic constraints seriously. After asking whether anyone else in the family could help out financially and finding out no one could, she asks whether Prudence's husband knows how angry she is. Prudence explains in great detail the ways she has tried to talk to him and the ways he refuses to hear her. Katherine questions whether Prudence's husband might respond differently if she told him that she was really having second thoughts about the marriage, and Prudence says, "He wouldn't. Believe me. He wouldn't." After a thorough exploration, divorce as a legitimate treatment option now seems closed.

Katherine proceeds by inquiring about other potentially oppositional options. She asks whether Prudence has ever "talked to any counselor type person." Prudence says that she has but infrequently. She has to take time off from work, and, as an hourly employee, she has the time deducted from her salary. Furthermore, her husband refuses to go to a therapist, does not want her to go either, and "knows every move I make." So getting regular therapeutic help would be difficult. This option, which might have helped her redefine her marriage, now also seems closed.

Katherine has explored with Prudence the possible treatment options of both a divorce and therapy, but neither seems feasible. Prudence does not want to end her marriage and, furthermore, cannot afford to. Nevertheless, Katherine raises the topic of divorce once again, and a struggle ensues in a social/ideological register. She asks, "Are you pretty clear that if the economics of the situation were different you would leave?", and Prudence responds by explaining that she is not sure.

> *N.P.* How long can you keep this up?
> *P.* I don't know because I am getting sick and tired of going to sleep early. It's been a long time.
> *N.P.* I suspect that's not the only way you're showing your anger. I suspect that other parts of your body are closing down as well. It's just not as easy for you to see. I'm really

concerned that this kind of strain over time will have a really negative effect on you. I absolutely understand that the economics of the situation, um, are their own problem. So that's why I was asking if the economics of the situation were taken care of, if that was out of the question, would you leave?

P. I don't know, I, I thought about it, but if it came right down to it, I don't know if I could . . .

N.P. Not right now anyway.

P. Yeah, probably not, not right now. I've been thinking about it. And it's getting more and more serious in my own mind, you know. At first, it's like, you know, just playing around with the idea. But it's getting more and more concrete as the time goes on. I just . . .

This is an interesting series of exchanges. Although Katherine repeatedly makes oppositional treatment recommendations and re-circulates the institutional authority associated with her professional status, she assiduously refrains from imposing either her medical expertise or her definition of the situation. Moreover, she has consistently avoided closure and resisted the temptation to medicalize Prudence's problems. Instead, she has engaged in a lengthy exploration of the social/biographical factors associated with Prudence's complaint of fatigue and suggested ways to treat it. In addition, whether as a medical provider or as a woman, she has persistently spoken in a social/ideological voice to articulate an oppositional discourse, averting both the definition of Prudence as overly emotional as well as traditional assumptions about women and the nuclear family. Yet, after posing divorce three times and therapy once as possible treatments, Katherine seems to change her approach.

In this exchange the nurse practitioner brings all the authority associated with her professional role to bear as she presses her definition of the situation—albeit an alternative one. She begins by asking Prudence how long she can continue to live in an untenable situation. Next, she tells her that being tired and falling asleep early are not the only ways she is showing her anger. "Other parts of your body are closing down as well." The image here is both unpleasant and frightening. Katherine continues by expressing her concern that the stress Prudence lives with "will over time have a really negative effect." From a medical provider, these messages take the form of a medical diagnosis and a treatment recommendation. As such, they carry a heavy load of cultural baggage. Since Katherine is not a friend and is a medical provider, she seeks the patient's compliance by relying on and recirculating both her professional status and the asymmetrical nature of the medical encounter. Prudence, however, resists and prevails.

There are striking similarities and equally dramatic differences in the way Katherine is communicating with Prudence and in the ways Doctor Aster talked with Wendy. Doctor Aster located Wendy's problem and defined the correct way to deal with it: Wendy is somatizing; the treatment is to stop working in the paid labor force so as to reduce the stress that is making her sick. Both the diagnosis and the treatment recommendation speak in a social/ideological voice and, in so doing, recirculate hegemonic assumptions about professional status and gendered identities.

Katherine is also speaking in a social/ideological voice and from her location as a medical expert. While she identifies Prudence's problem differently, she too defines the correct way to deal with it: Prudence, like Wendy, is making herself sick, somatizing. But where Wendy's emotions are out of control, Prudence's are legitimate. Her emotional response to an untenable situation makes her legitimately angry, and this anger produces her fatigue. Her problem is that she has not responded correctly. Katherine, like Doctor Aster, recommends the correct action to take. She recommends divorce, and she has recommended it now four times. The diagnosis, legitimate anger secondary to an untenable life situation, and the treatment recommendation, to get a divorce, while speaking in the voice of medicine, circulate both hegemonic and oppositional discourses. They reinscribe Katherine's professional status as the dominant interactional partner, and at the same time they resist and offer an alternative to dominant cultural assumptions about women, work, and the nuclear family.

While Doctor Aster's and Katherine's points of view are diametrically opposed, the similarity between this case and the previous one is overwhelming. Early in the encounter Doctor Aster identified the cause of Wendy's symptoms, and despite her resistance his definition of the problem remained consistent. Even though Prudence diagnoses herself and Katherine systematically legitimates this diagnosis, once Katherine defines divorce as the most appropriate treatment, she recommends it repeatedly. In this exchange, for example, while Katherine acknowledges that "the economics of the problem" are important, she asks, if they were taken care of, would Prudence act—would she get a divorce? Although Prudence has thought about divorce with increasing seriousness, she is consistent in her ambivalence.

This is not to say that there are not also significant differences in these cases. The disparity between a discourse that reinscribes hegemonic assumptions and one that is oppositional is certainly meaningful. The difference between an interaction that consistently positions the patient as incompetent and one that more often than not locates her as competent is also significant, as are the ways providers and patients struggle.

While in each case the patients resist and a struggle ensues in a social/ideological register, the outcomes are quite dissimilar. Although Wendy struggled with Doctor Aster's definition of the situation, the doctor systematically prevailed. By contrast, Prudence struggles both with herself and with Katherine's definition of the situation. The struggle with herself may be inconclusive. The struggle with Katherine has not been. Katherine has broached the subject of divorce four times and has suggested therapy once. She has used both her status as a medical provider and her location as a woman like Prudence to push for her definition of the situation, yet she has not been successful. Prudence has retained control. As far as she is concerned, therapy is not an option and neither, at this time, is divorce. Where Doctor Aster stuck to his definition of the situation despite Wendy's resistance, Katherine does not.

It is hard to know whether Katherine's next question picks up Prudence's frustration or her own.

N.P. What kinds of thoughts do you have about killing yourself?
P. Not many, I'm too chicken (Laughs.) I couldn't do it. (Laughs.) I'm scared of anything like that. I'm afraid of

dying, for that matter. I don't want to, you know. (Laughs.)
Besides that, I want to see my kids get older, and I want to be
there for their special moments, you know.

And a little later:

> *N.P.* Oftentimes, a man will try to take, to beat that out of
> a woman. Do you have any trouble with that?//
> *P.* //No, he's never, no, no. (Laughs.) If he ever did, I
> swear I'd do something when he was sleeping. (N.P. You
> would; laughs.) I would. I would never, uuh, you know, just
> do it. He knows I'm a very vengeful person when I want to
> be. No he's never hit me, never.

Although these are important questions and ones all too frequently
left unasked in medical encounters, they suggest that Prudence is
backed into a corner and that the relationship with her husband is
out of control—suggestions that are certainly warranted given the
preceding discussion. But here Prudence indicates that there is
something more than anger and frustration in her life, and this
something more has to do with her children. She also implies that
while she may be unhappy about her life and feel that she has no
options, she would not passively accept her husband's violence.

With these questions about the social/biographical context of
Prudence's life asked and answered, Katherine stops pushing her
treatment recommendations explicitly and begins the physical examination. Here, too, is an important distinction between the
nursing encounter and the medical consultation. Doctor Aster consistently avoided the social/biographical context of Wendy's life. In
addition, once he identified Wendy's problem in ideological terms
as social psychological, he largely abandoned medical topics and
medical care. For him the medical and the social seem to be separate areas, a diagnosis in one precludes an exploration in another.
Wendy, for example, had to tell Doctor Aster that she thought she
might be pregnant before he suggested a pregnancy test. And then
the test was performed more for social/ideological than medical
reasons, primarily to calm her fears rather than to determine whether
she was pregnant. This two-place logic is certainly not the case in

the nursing encounter. After a lengthy discussion of the social/biographical context of Prudence's life, Katherine does a comprehensive medical history and physical examination.

Turning her attention to the medical task at hand, Katherine asks about birth control and finds out that the patient has had her tubes tied. She then begins to take a medical history, focusing at first on stress-related problems. She asks Prudence what areas of her body she thinks are being harmed (a not-so-subtle reminder that she needs to take control of her life). When Prudence replies that she has no feeling that something is going wrong, Katherine asks about bowel health and about skin rashes. She takes Prudence's blood pressure and moves on to do a physical examination. She explains the importance of a yearly Pap smear and performs one on this visit. She does a breast examination, explains the importance of regular self-examinations, and teaches the patient how to examine her breasts. Finding the patient in essentially good health, she returns once more to the presenting complaint and the troubles in the patient's life, taking a different tone.

> *N.P.* One, one thing I would, I would, um, sort of, I don't want to use the word suggest because I, it's not that I think you *ought* to do it, consider. (P. Yeah.) One thing for you to *consider* is whether or not talking with your friends a (P. Yeah.) little more will help you to unload some of the feelings. I think there is sometimes a sense of loyalty or something that you don't want to wash all your dirty linens and so forth, and I absolutely understand that. I come from that tradition myself. The other side is you really have nothing to lose. (P. Yeah.) And, um, I suspect you're pretty good at figuring out which friends are trustworthy. (P. Yeah.) And I would encourage you to consider whether or not sharing a little more would help defuse some of the feelings. Yeah, it's not going to solve a whole lot, but, at least, it will diffuse some of the feelings and maybe help you to have some idea about how to go about things.
>
> *P.* Yeah, yeah. I have such a problem with dieting too. 'Cause when I get mad at him, I want to eat. Just to piss him off. I did so well. I had lost seventy pounds after I had Todd

[youngest child], and I pretty much kept it off. I want to lose a lot more, and I just, if I want . . . Another way I used to take out anger was I used to run—RUN RUN RUN RUN RUN—when I get angry. If I was real mad, oh God, I could go for miles (laughs) . . . But now he's just gotten to the point where he gets mad if I want to do that. You know, my God, he can't sit in the house for half an hour every night and watch the kids while I go out and run around the block. I'm not, you know, very far away. I'm just right around the block. And my girl friends and I were doing it, and he was getting . . . jealous because we had that half hour alone just to talk girl talk, you know. And he finally got so obnoxious about the whole thing, I just said forget it.

N.P. What would happen if you didn't say forget it?

P. Probably not much. I never thought of that. (Laughs.) Probably not much at all. He just, he'd just keep going. He's, he's like a little kid sometimes 'cause he sits there and pouts about it, you know.

N.P. Well it sounds to me that right now he is pouting no matter what you do. (P. Yeah.) So you might as well try doing things that will be good for you (P. Yeah.), and he can't do worse than he is doing right now.

P. Yeah . . . but I feel like a bad person sometimes when I do this. It's like "Oh God, how could I do this to him?" And then after I finally give in, I sit down and think, "How could he do this to me?" And I'm torn, you know? I don't know which way to turn.

N.P. I think one of the first big steps that I see going on in you now is that you are starting to pay more attention to yourself. (P. Yeah.) And I think that's gonna be your salvation. I think it's gonna bring the wrath of God down on you. (P. Yeah.) But it sounds to me as if the wrath of God is down on you anyway. (P. Yeah.) So even trying to cater to his needs, all you get is punished. So if you're gonna get punished, you might as well, at least, relieve some of your own needs at the same time.

P. Yeah, that's true. I never thought of that. I never thought of it.

N.P. I mean you might as well get punished for doing
something to get ahead, right? (Laughs.)

The discussion here is interesting. Katherine begins by saying that
she does not want to "suggest" how Prudence should deal with the
problems in her life. Instead, she wants to put forward some things
for Prudence to "*consider.*" This is a particularly fascinating formulation for two reasons. First, Katherine was much more forceful in her
earlier recommendations of divorce and therapy. This phrasing evi-
dences a real change in tone. Given the way she and Prudence
struggled over her prior treatment recommendations, it is hard to
know whether Katherine recognizes that she pushed hard, recirculating her institutional authority and her medical expertise in the process. However, it is clear that she does not do so here. Second, she
reframes and moderates her prior oppositional stand by making treatment recommendations that would allow Prudence to stay married
but to manage her anger and the symptoms associated with it effectively. And in each case she does so by producing a kind of symmetry
and one with no clear gender associations. This move toward a more
symmetrical relationship both relies on and distances Katherine from
the asymmetry characteristic of the provider-patient relationship.

Katherine asks Prudence to consider discussing her feelings with
her friends as a way to unload what she has been carrying around
inside of herself. Both asking the patient to consider a treatment
recommendation and the way Katherine frames her request do so-
cial/ideological work. She says, "I think there is sometimes a sense
of loyalty or something that you don't want to wash all your dirty
linens and so forth, and I absolutely understand that. *I come from
that tradition myself.*"[2]

Neither seeking the patient's considered agreement to a treatment nor disclosing this kind of personal information is common in
medical or nursing encounters. Providers usually just make recommendations and expect patients to follow them, with information
usually flowing from the person in authority (Goffman 1956, Jourard and Lasakow 1958, Brown 1965, Henley 1975, Fisher and
Groce 1990). In making this suggestion in this way, Katherine distances herself from her professional status. While in this instance
Katherine does not explicitly establish a solidarity based on their

common experiences as women, by talking person to person to Prudence and locating herself as a person, rather than a medical provider, she circulates a definition of herself as someone like Prudence. And then she marks this relationship by class. Like her, Prudence is a person of class who has reservations about airing her dirty linens in public.

From her professional position and after establishing that she is a person like Prudence, Katherine is able to subtly press her point of view and to garner Prudence's acceptance of it. She names Prudence's potential fears; then she affirms her. While people like Katherine and Prudence do not like to speak publicly about the less pleasant things in life, and while friends are not always trustworthy listeners, Katherine suspects that Prudence is "pretty good at figuring out which friends are trustworthy." Although she claims that talking to friends is not "going to solve a whole lot," Katherine strongly suggests that Prudence do what she can to defuse her feelings, which will help her decide how to proceed.

Prudence seems to agree; she says, "Yeah, yeah." Then she initiates a new topic: dieting. At first glance her response is unusual. Overwhelmingly, medical providers initiate topics and patients respond to them. Here, Prudence initiates a topic; however, the relationship between this topic and the prior discussion is hard to understand. It soon becomes clear. Talking more with friends is a specific suggestion within the larger topic of productive ways to deal with anger. When Prudence was dieting, she also ran, and running was a good way to manage her anger. But her husband objected. Even though she loved to run and knew it was good for her—good for both her diet and her anger—when her husband objected, she stopped. Prudence explains, "He finally got so obnoxious about the whole thing, I just said forget it."

In a social/ideological voice, Katherine asks a pointed question with an oppositional message. "What would happen if you didn't say forget it?" Implied in this question is another, and it too has an oppositional message: what would happen if you did not give in to your husband's "obnoxious" behavior, if you took care of yourself instead? While Prudence could not accept divorce or therapy as legitimate ways to deal with the problems in her life, the message here clearly makes more sense to her. She laughs and tells Katherine that "probably not much" would happen. She had not thought of it before, but her husband would probably just pout. Continuing in an oppositional vein, Katherine points out that since Prudence's husband seems to be pouting now and would pout if she ran regularly, she "might as well try doing things that will be good for you."

This message seems appealing to Prudence. She can stay married but work to redefine the marriage. But the choices still do not seem easy for her. Here we see how with Katherine's help she works her way through the conflict. Prudence first speaks the dominant cultural assumptions about men, women, and relationships as she names the fear that inhibits her ability to meet her needs. "I feel like a bad person. . . . How could I do this to him?" And then she speaks an oppositional discourse saying, "How could he do this to me?" She concludes that she feels torn and does not know where to turn. Katherine steps in and affirms Prudence's oppositional leanings. She affirms the big step Prudence is taking in paying more attention to herself, telling her it will be her "salvation." Although paying attention to herself will probably bring the wrath of God down on her, Katherine reminds her that "the wrath of God is down on you anyway. . . . So if you're gonna get punished, you might as well, at least, relieve some of your own needs at the same time." This support seems to help Prudence. "Yeah, that's true. I never thought of that. I never thought of it." Katherine laughs and makes her point again: "You might as well get punished for doing something to get ahead, right?"

Katherine and Prudence continue exploring ways Prudence can manage her problems, and throughout Katherine both speaks in a social/ideological voice and supports an oppositional discourse.

> *P.* It's true. I never thought of that. I never thought of it like that even when I told him. I got real obstinate with him. He got mad at me because I wanted out of the department. I wanted out of there and away from him. He said, "Well, who's gonna be my personal secretary?" 'Cause everybody that brings repairs over, and if he's not there, I have to take a message and give it to him. And I don't want to do it anymore. I was so mad, I told him, "You take your own damn messages." He was just so upset about it, and I said, "I don't give a shit!" That's just what I told him.
>
> *N.P.* Good for you!

P. For three days he barely talked to me, but he's gotten better about it.

N.P. I was gonna say, he survived, right?

P. Yeah, he survived.

N.P. So that gives you a lesson, right?

P. He's feeling a lot better about it now.

N.P. Well, I think the two things that you might consider first, and I know you already are, the business at work . . . getting your job changed (P. Yeah.) because I think you're absolutely right. I think that's a real essential pursuit . . .

P. //Yeah, it just hit me a few weeks ago. Something told me to get out of there.

N.P. Right. The second thing is to pick something, and it sounds like running may be the something because it would solve a couple of problems. First of all it would get you out (P. Yeah.) and it would be wonderful; and it would also let you pound your anger into the pavement (P. Yeah.) or the dirt or whatever . . . One thing about running is that the actual exercise, um, helps with depression. It physiologically releases an enzyme that helps with depression. (P. Wow; laughs.) So that it will help your energy level in addition to everything else (P. Yeah.), and if it's something you love to do and it feels good to you, I would, I can't tell you how strongly I would recommend that be one of the places you, you set up that you're not gonna give up. (P. I love it!) That this is your thing that you're not going to give up. Then you can do it every day.

P. I love to run. I would more or less jog every day.

N.P. Exactly!

We can almost hear Prudence coming to the realization that she can stay married but resist her husband and withstand the "obnoxious" behavior that in all probability will result. She talks about wanting to change jobs so that she does not work next to him and is not expected to act as his personal secretary. She remembers aloud her husband's anger when she refused to meet these expectations. But she did not give in. Katherine supports her vigorously. "Good for you!" Prudence continues as if thinking aloud. She explains that although her husband was angry and barely talked to her, he got over it. Katherine brings the point sharply into focus. "He survived, right?" And when Prudence agrees, she continues, "So that gives you a lesson, right?" Katherine, speaking in a social/ideological voice and circulating an oppositional discourse, sums up the treatment recommendations. Prudence should continue trying to change her job, and she should continue to run.

It is interesting that while talking about the social/biographical context of Prudence's life, Katherine only uses the power associated with her professional status twice. Both times she is recommending a way to treat Prudence's anger and the fatigue that results from it. When discussing divorce for the fourth time and in the face of continued resistance by Prudence, Katherine brings all the authority or her medical expertise to bear. She speaks in vague but dire terms about the health risks of unmediated anger. Now she once again brings her medical expertise to bear, but this time she does so to bring home the health benefits of running. Not only would running get Prudence out of the house and let her pound her anger into the pavement, but it is an effective treatment for depression as well. "It physiologically releases an enzyme that helps with depression." Where Prudence resisted the earlier treatment recommendations, she does not reject this one. Quite the contrary. Prudence says, "I love to run. I would more or less jog every day." And Katherine responds, "Exactly!"

Katherine and Prudence have reached a diagnosis and an agreement about treatment. Earlier, Prudence positions her struggle in two different conflicts—one between marriage and divorce and another about how to define or redefine her marriage. When Katherine and Prudence discuss divorce and therapy as potential treatments, their deliberation is marked by a struggle in which Prudence prevails. In the discussion about how to redefine Prudence's marriage, there is no similar struggle. After some initial resistance, Katherine helps Prudence work her way through conflicting ways to be married. Then they agree that talking more with friends, running, and changing jobs are all potentially good strategies for both staying married and dealing with Prudence's fatigue. In fact, Prudence initiates two of the topics that become treatment recommendations—running and changing jobs.

For several reasons this consultation is particularly striking. Unlike Doctor Aster, Katherine does not bring all the authority of her medical role to bear in defining the patient as incompetent, in limiting the discussion to the issues she defines as legitimate, or in revivifying her professional status or the patient's gendered identity. Instead, she asks questions and follows through on the patient's answers. By probing to get additional information, Katherine provides the space for Prudence to tell her story and display her competence. In fact, Katherine facilitates this storytelling, which is done in a social/biographical register.

Katherine certainly seems to be providing just the kind of care that Mishler (1984) and other reformers call for—care that minimizes the asymmetry of the medical relationship and maximizes the voice of the patient's lifeworld. However, the inclusion of a discourse about the social/biographical context of Prudence's life does not seem to terminate the institutional authority of the provider. When seeking the patient's compliance to the first treatment she recommends, Katherine takes control. She speaks an oppositional discourse, and when this is not successful, she brings all the authority of her medical expertise to bear; a struggle ensues in a social/ideological register—a struggle in which at first the patient prevails. Prudence successfully resists Katherine's recommendation of divorce and only later agrees to the compromise recommendation of talking with friends and running.

The tension here between conflicting positions is particularly interesting. Both provider and patient seem to be caught between conflicting positions, although different ones. From the beginning of this encounter and throughout, Prudence speaks about her life, and as she speaks she makes visible tensions between traditional and alternative discourses about women, work, and the nuclear family. While these conflicts produce a struggle for her, they produces no similar struggle for the nurse practitioner. Whether speaking as a professional or as a woman like Prudence, Katherine consistently speaks and supports an oppositional discourse. In Prudence's conflict between staying married and getting divorced, she comes down firmly on the side of divorce. And in the conflict between a more and less traditional marriage, she staunchly supports a less traditional, more egalitarian relationship in which Prudence can pay attention to her own needs.

As a medical provider Katherine too is caught between discourses—between the disparity of provider and patient in the medical encounter and their solidarity as women of a certain class. Katherine relies on and recirculates the characteristic asymmetry of the provider-patient relationship. She encourages and incites Prudence to speak a discourse of the social, and she does so without limiting the discussion to the narrowly defined parameters of the patient's domestic arrangements. And this social talk does not so totally define the encounter that medical topics are abandoned. The nurse practitioner seems to move easily from a discussion of Prudence's life to the traditional medical history and physical examination. But, whether speaking in a social or a medical voice, when Katherine seeks Prudence's compliance to the treatments she has recommended, she brings all the authority usually associated with her professional status to bear and does so in ways that are deeply ideological and political. Prudence at first resists successfully; however, in the end the provider prevails, and they reach a compromise agreement. Social and medical voices certainly seem to interrupt and interpenetrate each other in ways they did not in the medical consultation; however, they are more complex than they might at first seem to be, and neither voice automatically erases the institutional authority so characteristic of the medical relationship.

Katherine both relies on and distances herself from this asymmetry to produce and maintain discourses of solidarity. She works to locate herself as a woman like Prudence, to produce and maintain a gender solidarity based in women's common experiences. And she works to locate Prudence as a woman like herself, a woman with whom she shares a code of etiquette; in so doing, she produces and maintains a solidarity based on class. While the nurse practitioner sets the discursive mode here, these interactions no longer support a two-place logic in which the provider is dominant and competent and the patient is neither. However, they also do not completely erase these differences. It appears, then, that this consultation both recirculates the asymmetry usually associated with the provider-patient relationship and offers an alternative to it.

FIVE

COMPLAINTS CODED
AS MEDICAL
The Medical Consultation

The discourse of the social that Mishler (1984) and other reformers call for and the caring that nurse practitioners claim to provide rely on a distinction between talk that is about medical topics and talk that is more social psychological in nature—a distinction that both Waitzkin (1983) and Silverman (1987) criticize and one that is problematic in the cases just discussed. In the nursing and medical consultations I discuss in Chapters Three and Four, the social penetrates presumably medical discussions, and the relationship between the social and the medical is more complex than it might at first appear to be.

Yet these cases may offer a special opportunity for social and medical voices to interrupt and interpenetrate each other. Both encounters lend themselves to being marked as social psychological rather than medical in nature. This coding is representative of the larger corpus of material and provides an opportunity to illuminate persistent patterns. However, both the coding and the ways social and medical discourses function raise important questions. Does labeling a presenting complaint social psychological rather than medical pave the way for a more social discourse? Do patients whose life stories locate them at an intersection between traditional and alternative discourses about women, work, and the nuclear family provide an especially fertile opportunity for a discourse of the social? Without a comparison we could conclude that the nature of the complaint, the status of the patients as young, married mothers working in the paid labor force, the lives of these patients, or all three factors account for the character of the discourse.

There is another equally pressing question about whether medicine and nursing provide essentially different sites for the production of knowledge, the negotiation of identity, and the delivery of care. Despite the similarities in the cases just discussed, there seem to be significant distinctions, which comparisons also could clarify. While Doctor Aster and Wendy struggle in a social/ideological register over competing definitions of her medical complaint—definitions that are firmly situated in the social/biographical context of her life—the doctor's position consistently prevails. Notwithstanding Wendy's resistance, hegemonic assumptions about the appropriate behavior for men and women are insistently reinscribed. In this process an asymmetrical medical relationship, with a dominant doctor and a subordinate patient, is just as persistently revivified.

In some ways the nursing consultation seems less clear cut. Here too provider and patient struggle over competing social/ideological discourses about the nuclear family and the provider-patient relationship. But although the nurse practitioner solicits information about the social/biographical context of the patient's life and the doctor does not, Katherine's definition of the situation and her treatment recommendation do not always prevail but Doctor Aster's do. On several occasions Prudence resists and does so successfully. In addition, Katherine both reenacts the asymmetry of the provider-patient relationship and distances herself from it. By locating herself as a woman like Prudence and situating Prudence as a person who shares her class position, Katherine moves to minimize the distance between provider and patient. Nevertheless, Katherine has the last word. In the end, whether speaking as a provider or speaking as a person like Prudence, her definitions prevail. One aspect of the nursing consultation is clearly handled in a dramatically different way than it is in the medical consultation. Where at every opportunity Doctor Aster insistently reinscribes hegemonic assumptions about women and family, Katherine does not. Quite the contrary. From the beginning of the nursing encounter and throughout it, Katherine consistently speaks an oppositional discourse.

These similarities and differences raise important questions about the nature of the medical and nursing consultations. To begin to address these issues, I chose two additional cases—and I chose them for their comparability and their potential contrasts. As in the prior cases, Doctor Johnson and Claudia Sussen, the nurse practitioner, are primary-care providers who share a commitment to patient-centered holistic medicine, which integrates the medical and the social. The stated intentions, then, of all the providers are quite similar. Moreover, each of the providers practices in a primary-care setting. Both doctors practice in a model family-practice clinic associated with a teaching hospital, while both nurse practitioners provide care in neighborhood clinics with strong ties to a university school of nursing. Each setting, then, has a double mission—to provide high-quality, cost-effective primary care and to train future providers. Finally, the patients, Muriel Whales and Pat Scott, like the prior two patients, are both women.

Here the comparability among these cases ends and the contrasts begin. The first contrasts are between age, class, and social location. Unlike the prior patients, Muriel and Pat are not working-to-middle class. Neither are they young women struggling with the conflicting demands of a nuclear family and a position in the paid labor force. At the time of their medical consultations, Muriel and Pat are neither living in a nuclear family nor employed in the paid labor force. Both women are middle-aged—forty-five and fifty-four, respectively. They are both poor, single heads of households. Muriel is a Caucasian woman living in rural Appalachia. She is recently widowed and the mother of seven children ranging from thirteen to twenty-seven years old. Four of her teenage children and two grandchildren are currently living in a trailer with her. Pat is an urban African American woman. After living in a nuclear family, she is, by the time of this interview, living alone and isolated. Her child is grown, and her mate has left.

In addition, these cases provide a contrast between initial visits and routine care and between urgent and chronic medical problems. Doctor Aster and Katherine Heinz are seeing Wendy and Prudence for the first time, and each patient presents with an urgent complaint. While Muriel's visit with Doctor Johnson is an initial one for an urgent problem, Pat's visit with Claudia Sussen is a routine one for a chronic problem.

Moreover, the nature of the patients' presenting complaints is quite different. Just as Wendy's and Prudence's presenting complaints are easily marked as psychosomatic, Muriel's and Pat's are just as easily coded as medical. Muriel, who had a hysterectomy seven years ago, has had intermittent vaginal bleeding, and Pat, who is a diabetic and has high blood pressure, presents with a scab on her arm that will not clear up. Both complaints could be serious. Vaginal bleeding in a woman who no longer menstruates could be a sign of cancer, and infections are potentially life-threatening for diabetics.

While these cases, like the previous two, are representative of the larger corpus of material from which they are drawn and provide similar opportunities to illuminate persistent patterns, they also offer important points of comparison. Since these complaints cannot easily be marked as psychosomatic and since neither of these patients is a young woman living at the juncture between traditional and alternative discourses about women, work, and the nuclear family, these consultations allow us to decide whether the previous cases provided especially fertile sites for the production of social discourses and, if so, how. Furthermore in the present cases class and race more explicitly enter the interactional equation, and these factors also may effect the ways provider and patient communicate. They thereby provide an expanded opportunity to explore how race, class, gender, and age intersect in both the production of meaning and the way health care is delivered. There is an additional opportunity here as well. If social discourses have penetrated these consultations, comparing the ways the social is struggled over and exploring the ideological effects of these struggles set the stage for the analysis in subsequent chapters.

In Chapters Five and Six, as in Chapters Three and Four, I examine two transcripts in depth—one with a doctor and a woman patient and another with a nurse practitioner and a woman patient. In each I look for recurrent patterns in form—the discourse structure —and in the content of the communication and analyze the ideological work done as provider and patient talk with each other.

The medical consultation begins with Doctor Johnson walking into an examining room where the patient, Muriel Whales, is waiting. She is Caucasian, and, although only forty-five, she looks old and worn. To anyone familiar with the region, she is easy to identify as a poor, rural, Appalachian woman—an identification verified in the medical file the doctor holds as he enters the examining room. Doctor Johnson is a young, Caucasian man who also is easily identified as an Appalachian, although he is clearly not now poor.

The consultation begins with Muriel sitting on the examining table clothed in only a paper hospital gown. Even so, she carries the marks of her identity. She is older, overweight, clean but shabby, and not very well groomed. Doctor Johnson enters the examining room dressed in street clothes and wearing the marks of his professional status—a white coat and a stethoscope.[1] He remains standing, looks down on the patient, and without introducing himself greets her. Even though the greeting takes an everyday form, it has not occurred in an everyday setting. It takes place in a medical setting and in the face of subtle cues that have already located doctor and patient and established the status differences between them.

> *D.* Well, hello, ma'am. How have you been?
> *P.* Not too good.

The doctor's everyday greeting produces an everyday response but not a presenting complaint. Dr. Johnson tries again.

> *D.* Well, what can I do to help you then?
> *P.* The last three or four months I've had . . . (D. Uh hum.) a hysterectomy about seven years ago (D. I see.); and now I saw a period, and it's not light. It's real dark.
> *D.* I'm sorry, what did you say you had done to you seven years ago?
> *P.* I had a hysterectomy.
> *D.* You had your uterus taken out. Is that correct?
> *P.* (Nods in the affirmative.)
> *D.* Now tell me about the bleeding you're having now, ma'am?
> *P.* That's what I'm saying. I've started, and I don't know where it's coming from, and I don't know what's causing it, whether it's nerves or what it is; and when I do this I'm real, real sick. I'm sick at my stomach, and I just wanna throw up.

And here lately, for the last two or three months, I've been real, real nervous.

There is a lot going on in these opening interactions. While at first glance they seem both familiar and innocuous, from the opening moment of the consultation and throughout it, social assumptions are penetrating a discussion that is presumably about a medical complaint. While some of these assumptions are subtle and some are not, and some are verbal and others are not, they do ideological work.

While Doctor Johnson does not introduce himself, greet the patient by name, or ask what the problem is, Muriel does not challenge him. Quite the contrary. She follows his lead. If he issues an everyday greeting, she responds in kind. When he switches to a more medical frame, she follows suit. Muriel starts to explain that for the last three or four months she has had, she pauses slightly, and the doctor urges her to continue with his back channel comment, "Uh hum." She starts again further back in her story. She had a hysterectomy seven years ago and now she unmistakably has seen what she identifies as menstrual blood—"real dark."

Perhaps the shift from the present time frame—the last three or four months—to one further back in time—seven years ago—confuses the doctor. Perhaps he is confused by her presentation of an impossible set of medical facts—a hysterectomy seven years ago and a menstrual period now. In either case, he apologizes and asks her to repeat what had been done to her seven years ago. Her response, "I had a hysterectomy," is clear and unambiguous, yet the doctor checks further. "You had your uterus taken out. Is that correct?" While a hysterectomy may need further clarification, it is not usually of this kind. A doctor might need to know whether just the uterus or both the uterus and ovaries were removed. But Doctor Johnson does not clarify in this way. Instead he challenges the information Muriel has provided by exploring whether Muriel understands that a hysterectomy is the surgical removal of the uterus. And, in so doing, he suggests that a woman like Muriel—a poor woman—neither understands medical terminology nor is a competent, trustworthy reporter of her medical history. This suggestion carries clear class and gender implications. Imagine a doctor checking in a similar way to see whether a middle-class woman correctly remembers that she has had a hysterectomy and understands that her uterus was removed in the surgery. It is even harder to imagine a doctor questioning a man about whether he understands that his prostate gland was surgically removed by a prostatectomy.

These exchanges do social/ideological work. While at first glance doctor and patient may seem like equal interactional partners, that impression quickly fades. At first, Doctor Johnson seems deferential. He calls the patient "ma'am" and apologizes for asking her to repeat herself. However, the doctor opens the consultation, directs the discussion of topics, and checks to see whether the patient knows what she is talking about. In the process he recirculates dominant cultural assumptions about the medical relationship and the relative positions of doctor and patient in it. In this opening sequence, then, medical topics are discussed as identities are negotiated.

After confirming that Muriel understands that her uterus was surgically removed seven years ago, Doctor Johnson asks her to tell him about the bleeding. Muriel may be poor and is probably uneducated, but she certainly seems to pick up and be annoyed by how hard it is to establish her presenting complaint. She says, "That's what I'm saying," and then elaborates on why she is there. She does not know where the bleeding is coming from or what is causing it, but it is accompanied by being sick to her stomach. She then adds that she has been nervous for the last two or three months.

These are interesting exchanges. By being annoyed that Doctor Johnson has treated her as a less-than-competent reporter of her medical history, Muriel subtly resists the doctor's social/ideological definition of the situation and makes visible a competing discourse about poor women in which they are competent to tell their medical stories. This presentation both repositions Muriel and undermines the asymmetry characteristic of the medical relationship. But she does not prevail.

Doctor Johnson does not seem to notice her annoyance and continues to pay selective attention to what she has to say. As the discussion continues, she expands on her presenting complaint. She links vaginal bleeding to feeling sick and specifies how she feels sick.

"I'm sick at my stomach, and I just wanna throw up." And then she connects both symptoms to a social/biographical origin. She states that she does not know whether the bleeding is coming from nerves, but she has been "real, real nervous." Doctor Johnson follows through neither on her medical symptom—feeling sick to her stomach—nor on her more social/biographical explanations, which tie her physical symptoms to the stressful context of her everyday life. Instead he continues by following a narrow and ideologically defined medical story line.

> D. How much bleeding are we talking about?
> P. Uh, it messes up my clothes, and I have to change clothes two or three times a day.
> D. Does it cause little spots on your panties or on your slacks?
> P. On my panties.
> D. On your panties. Okay.
> P. And it's done sometimes at night, more or less at night, sometimes at daytime.
> D. Uh, hum, and how long does it last when it starts?
> P. Sometimes it lasts three or four days; then sometimes it comes and goes.
> D. Have you been doing anything to stop it?
> P. No.
> D. Have you noticed anything that makes it worse?
> P. No.
> D. Okay, prior to, now when did you say this started? I'm sorry.
> P. About three months ago.
> D. Prior to three months ago, had you had any problems with vaginal bleeding since you had your uterus taken out?
> P. (Nods no.)
> D. None whatsoever?

Once again while medical topics are being discussed, social/ideological work is being done. At first glance the information exchanged may not seem problematic. Doctor Johnson asks, "How

much bleeding are we talking about?" On its surface this is an inno-
cent question, but it carries strong social/ideological overtones.
While asking for medical information, it simultaneously implies
that Muriel may not be reporting her symptoms accurately. She
may be exaggerating the amount of bleeding or responding in an
overly emotional way to a little bit of blood. Her identity as an
overly emotional woman or as an incompetent reporter of her medical history (or both) is thus being produced.

Bleeding after a hysterectomy, whether in small or large
amounts, is one of the primary warning signs of cancer and is,
therefore, something to be concerned about. Yet Doctor Johnson
does not treat this medical information seriously. He does not take a
fuller medical history to explore other changes that might be associated with cancer. He does not ask her, for example, to talk more
about the relationship she has reported between nausea and bleeding or whether she has noticed any changes in her bowels.

While Doctor Johnson's challenge carries a clear message—a so-
cial/ideological message with class and gender implications—it is in
other respects an empty question. He uses it neither to address the
medical facts associated with this symptom nor to explore other
social/biographical topics connected to it. He does not question
what might have changed in Muriel's life or her behavior recently.
Perhaps she is engaging in rough sex. Perhaps she has a vaginal
infection or a sexually transmitted disease. Nor does he inquire
about the relationship Muriel has reported between the bleeding
and being nervous. He does not ask how the patient is making sense
of her symptoms. He asks neither whether the symptoms she has
reported are making her nervous nor what she imagines them to
indicate.

In other words, the doctor does not question whether a medical
discourse about this kind of bleeding has entered Muriel's own account of herself—whether she may be interpreting her symptoms
in light of a cultural discourse about women and cancer. These silences—the questions not asked—do social/ideological work. They
present Muriel as an overly emotional woman and an incompetent
patient, and they deny her membership in a common culture in
which these symptoms are widely recognized as a potential indica-

tion of cancer. And they also foreclose potential discussions of relevant medical and social/biographical topics.

Instead, Doctor Johnson challenges Muriel's responses. The patient has told him that the bleeding is heavy enough so that she has to change her clothes two or three times a day. While it might have been necessary for Doctor Johnson to establish the medical facts— whether the clothes were soaked with blood or whether the blood just stained her underwear—he does not do so. He asks a medical sounding question—"Does it cause little spots on your panties or on your slacks?" In medical terms this is another empty question. Any bleeding in a woman who has had a hysterectomy is significant. But from a social/ideological perspective it is certainly not empty. It trivializes the patient's claim that the bleeding is significant enough to have her change her clothes several times a day—significant enough to warrant a medical examination. It also sends a more subtle social/ideological message that again has strong class and gender associations—a consistent message that presents her as an overly emotional woman and an incompetent patient. Again, the message emerges most clearly by comparison. Imagine a doctor asking a man complaining of penile bleeding whether his panties were stained. More subtle still is the assumption that she routinely wears slacks. Poor rural Appalachians work the land, and this work is rarely done in a dress.

Doctor Johnson then asks for the medical facts yet again and apologizes for the repetition: "When did you say this started. I'm sorry." Muriel's responses have now established clearly that the bleeding is both a fairly recent change and sporadic. Nevertheless, he checks again. He asks her whether from the time her uterus was removed to three months ago she had problems with vaginal bleeding. Muriel shakes her head no. He has asked a question and gotten a clear response. But the doctor asks for further confirmation about the lack of bleeding prior to three months ago: "None whatsoever?" Doctor Johnson has now challenged Muriel's competence to accurately report her symptoms three times and she has consistently demonstrated that she knows what she is talking about.

The questions asked and those not asked again do both medical and social/ideological work. While Doctor Johnson fails to gather the kind of information that would allow him to diagnose and treat Muriel's medical problem or to allay her fears, he does consistently reproduce his professional status as the dominant interactional partner and thereby reinscribes the asymmetry of the medical relationship. From this dominant position, he avoids Muriel's social/biographical cues with his focused and ideologically loaded medical questions, trivializes her presenting complaint, implies she may be exaggerating her bleeding, demeans her status as a competent patient, and denies her membership in a common culture. He repeatedly treats her as a poor, uneducated woman who is both overly emotional and unable to understand or accurately report on a complex medical phenomenon. In this way he persistently reproduces her identity as a lower-class woman patient and recirculates dominant social/ideological assumptions about class and gender.

While Muriel does not explicitly resist Doctor Johnson's definition of the situation, she does struggle against it, and these struggles occur in a social/ideological register. She demonstrates that she understands what a hysterectomy is, has had one, and, nevertheless, is experiencing repeated episodes of vaginal bleeding. In so doing she depicts herself as a competent patient with sound emotions and struggles against the asymmetrical nature of the medical relationship as well as the doctor's authority to define. But to no avail. At every opportunity Doctor Johnson reiterates his definition of the situation and, despite her struggle, reproduces it.

It is tempting to conclude that Doctor Johnson is a poorly trained physician, lacking essential social and medical skills; however, interactions of this kind are too common, too familiar, and too insidious for such individualistic conclusions to suffice. Moreover, these interactions can be seen as successful. While verifying the presenting complaint—a medical topic—the participants have negotiated their identities as doctor and patient, man and woman. This social/ideological work consistently reproduces dominant cultural assumptions, and it continues to do so in subsequent interactions.

The consultation continues as Doctor Johnson begins to take a social and medical history. This section of the discussion wanders through several pages of the transcript. Through a series of rambling questions a picture of Muriel's life emerges. Her father died two years ago, and her husband died shortly thereafter. She lives with four children and two grandchildren in a trailer. One of these children, her eighteen-year-old daughter, is pregnant. As she describes her life, her nervousness is easy to understand. It could easily be related to her family situation. Doctor Johnson again listens selectively. Since these life conditions cannot account for Muriel's bleeding, he pursues them no further. This lack of attention to the social/biographical context of Muriel's life both trivializes it and defines what is and is not a legitimate topic of discussion.

After taking a limited social history, Doctor Johnson returns to a medical topic. He asks a few rather standard questions. Do you wear glasses? Any changes in your hearing? Bothered much by sore throats?[2] He then begins the physical examination. While doing the exam, he continues to ask questions usually asked while taking a medical history.

> *D.* Now you tell me if I hurt you. Is it tender right here [stomach]?
> *P.* Yeah.
> *D.* How about over on that side?
> *P.* No, not right there.

He continues to palpate her stomach.

> *D.* You noticed any changes in your weight recently?
> *P.* (Nods yes.)
> *D.* In what way?
> *P.* Because I know I'm overweight, yip, very overweight.
> *D.* Uh huh, has it gotten worse lately? Have you gained a whole lot of weight lately, or have you lost any weight recently?
> *P.* I think I lost a little bit.
> *D.* Okay. Do you remember how much you weighed last time you were weighed before today, or has it been so long ago that you don't remember?
> *P.* Well, they weighed me back about a month ago, and I don't know how much I weighed.

Still later in the exam the doctor returns to the medical history.

D. Do you have diarrhea or constipation?
P. No.
D. When was the last time you were constipated?
P. I don't know.
D. Longer than a year, longer than three years?
P. I really don't know.

Each of these questions is important in establishing a differential diagnosis. Questioning whether the patient experiences pain in her abdomen on palpation and whether she has noticed changes in her weight or in her bowels is especially important if one has concerns about cancer. However, while these questions reproduce consistent social/ideological assumptions, they are not asked, for the most part, in ways that would elicit the fullest medical response.

The question about pain on palpation of the abdomen can reasonably be asked only during the physical exam. However, the second question, about changes in the patient's weight, lacks sensitivity. It is probably unproductive to ask an overweight woman questions about her weight while manually probing her stomach. In a society that values slenderness, especially for women, it is hard to imagine an overweight woman who would not be self-protective when asked in this way. The location of the question during the physical exam, then, seems to frame the response. If this is an important question for the diagnosis, the doctor might have received a more useful response if he had asked it while taking a medical history.

Similarly, the doctor might have obtained more information if he had asked whether there had been changes in bowel habits recently. After the patient responded to that question, he might have probed with more specific questions about diarrhea and constipation. As asked, his question is not likely to produce the information he is seeking. Unless one has chronic problems with bowels, the response to the question "Do you have diarrhea or constipation?" would most likely be no.

While the doctor's questions about weight and bowel habits are not skillful in eliciting medical information, they send social/ideological messages that by now are all too familiar. Once again Doctor Johnson challenges the information Muriel has provided. His first question—"Do you remember how much you weighed last time you were weighed before today, or has it been so long that you don't remember?"—seems reasonable. Surely an overweight woman who has recently lost weight would remember when she was weighed and how much weight she had lost. However, if she does not remember, her claim that she has lost a little weight will be invalidated, and she will appear incompetent. And that is just what happens. Muriel responds by explaining that even though she was weighed just last month, she does not remember how much she weighed.

Doctor Johnson's questions about constipation produce similar results. Muriel has said she has not had either diarrhea or constipation. And again the doctor challenges her answer by pressing for specific information. "Longer than a year, longer than three years?" Since Muriel has only been bleeding for three months, these questions also make little sense medically, but they send a consistent social/ideological message: by implication, others, presumably more competent others, would be able to provide answers. Since Muriel is unable to do so, she is clearly not competent. However, probably no one who neither is plagued by recurrent bouts of constipation or diarrhea nor has had a recent episode could have answered these questions any better.

It is all too easy to connect Muriel's presumed incompetence with both her gender and her class and thus to reinscribe the notion that both lower-class people and women are different, are "less than." This difference is established by its implied contrast to "normal" people. Normal people are competent, but women and lower-class people are not. You cannot trust them to be able to tell you the truth about their lives. During a presumably medical discussion Doctor Johnson has been sending this ideological message consistently, and for the most part Muriel has not resisted.

The doctor continues his physical examination by asking the patient to lie down, to scoot all the way down on the table, to let her legs go wide apart, and to let this muscle here (touching the vaginal opening) go nice and easy. With these instructions he begins to do a vaginal exam.

D. You're a very wet person.
P. Uh uh.

He then finishes his examination:

D. Okay, just go ahead and lean back here, scoot
backwards. You can go ahead and sit up, Miss Whales. Okay,
Miss Whales, I took two specimens. Okay, I took one which
we call a wet prep, and I'm going to take it to the microscope
right now, which will tell us if you have any local irritation,
infections. Okay, the other specimen I took for a Pap smear.
Okay, even though you've had your uterus taken out you
need to have a Pap smear about every year. Okay.
P. Okay.

In the context of the patient's presenting complaint both a Pap
smear and a wet prep make sense. In the absence of a uterus, the
Pap smear checks for vaginal cancer and the wet prep for certain
kinds of vaginal infections. But while these tests may be necessary,
they are probably not sufficient. The doctor has not taken a comprehensive medical history. And he has taken no sexual history. He
has not even asked Muriel whether she is sexually active and treats
her as if she were not. In a population where sexually transmitted
diseases are at epidemic proportions, he does not perform the appropriate procedures to test for them.

As the doctor begins this exam, he gives Muriel behavioral directions. Although they are sometimes given with more finesse, these
are not uncommon directions. It is, however, uncommon to perform procedures without first explaining them and asking the patient's permission to proceed.

But even more uncommon is the doctor's next comment, "You're
a very wet person." Not only is it uncommon, but it is also uncalled
for and uncouth. Vaginal wetness is usually associated with sexual
stimulation. Is he implying that Muriel is sexually stimulated? By
him? By the exam? Such a response is not only inappropriate in a
medical situation, but it opens an ideological can of worms. Inappropriate sexual responses—responses that break societal norms—
are often attributed to loose women of the lower classes. Is he im-

plying that Muriel is such a woman? Women's sexuality is often seen as dirty. Is he implying that Muriel is an unmarried, lower-class, dirty, sexually stimulated woman? Whatever he is implying, this is not just a neutral observation done in the objective voice of medicine. It is an ideological comment masquerading as a medical observation.

Here, cultural assumptions have structured how information is and is not exchanged. It could be argued that the doctor does not take a sexual history because he assumes that an older woman whose husband is recently deceased is not sexually active. Such an assumption would recirculate traditional notions about women, age, sexuality, and domestic relations. It would also be at odds with Doctor Johnson's finding of vaginal wetness. If he has assumed that sexual stimulation goes with marriage or that older women are neither sexually stimulated nor sexually active, finding vaginal lubrication on physical examination would position Muriel as out of sync with these assumptions. This finding may have surprised the doctor, and his surprise may account for his comment.

However, both the assumption that Muriel has recently lost her husband and, thus, is no longer sexually active and the assumption that vaginal wetness signals an active sexuality and is inappropriate for an older, recently widowed woman send messages about the appropriate way to be a sexually active woman. They also send messages about the professional status of the doctor. Muriel does not resist either message. Moreover, she does not take the doctor to task for his inappropriate statement. Her not doing so contributes to the reproduction of their respective identities—his as the all-knowing doctor and hers as a lower-class, sexually inappropriate woman.

With the physical examination concluded, Doctor Johnson again gives Muriel behavioral directions, calling her *Miss* Whales." In light of the earlier messages he has sent, this is a particularly interesting exchange. Speaking in the voice of medicine, the doctor circulates subtle social/ideological messages. By referring to Muriel as Miss Whales, he erases her marital status, relocates her as a single woman, and subtly fortifies the impression that she is somehow sexually inappropriate. After this exchange Doctor Johnson leaves the examining room, and I leave with him.

For several reasons this has been a difficult consultation for me to observe. While presumably discussing medical topics, Doctor Johnson has consistently spoken a social/ideological discourse that undermines Muriel's status as a good woman, and, in addition, he has left important medical topics unaddressed. The patient has dropped hints indicating that she is aware of a discourse linking the kind of bleeding she has been having with cancer. I suspect that she thinks she has cancer, and that is what has brought her to see the doctor. I am disturbed that Doctor Johnson has not addressed this fear with her. I am also troubled because I do not feel the doctor has taken an adequate history or performed all the necessary tests. For example, he has not found out why Muriel had a hysterectomy. Perhaps she had cancer earlier. If so, that could be important information for him to have. Neither has he taken a sexual history. Although one of the slides he makes is to check for a vaginal infection, certainly a sexual history and a gonorrhea culture are also called for.

Since my position in this setting is as both a researcher and a teacher,[3] I can address my concerns with the doctor, and I do. I point out that he has not found out why the hysterectomy was done in the first place, and then I share my observation that the patient seems concerned that she may have cancer. He has not considered either possibility. He tells me that while he cannot be certain, on both visual and manual examination it does not look like cancer. He thinks it much more likely that it is some kind of infection or irritation. I hold my tongue and do not ask him why he has not shared this observation with the patient. Instead, I suggest that when he returns to the examining room he find out why the patient has had a hysterectomy and reassure her that he does not think she has cancer now.

I continue by telling him that I am confused about why he has not taken a sexual history or done a gonorrhea culture. He looks confused by my confusion and says, "She's forty-five years old, and her husband has only been dead for twenty months." I then ask if he is assuming that she is not sexually active, and he says yes. This time I cannot hold my tongue. I tell him that I am forty-five years old and that I can attest to the fact that women do not automatically lose their sexual interest at some magic age, whether single or married.[4] I suggest that, rather than assuming Muriel is sexually inactive, he ask her. When he returns to the examining room, our discussion is reflected in the conversation.

D. Okay. Mrs. Whales, a couple of things I neglected to ask you earlier that are relevant to what's going on. Okay, first, why did you have your uterus removed seven years ago?

P. Ah, because, ah, my period it would, it came and it wouldn't stop.

D. Uh, how long would it last?

P. A whole month.

D. Okay, so you had a period of time where you were bleeding for up to a month (P. Um hum.), and that's why they took your uterus out.

P. And at the time, too, I was on birth-control pills, and when I got pregnant with my last little girl, I cried for four days because I didn't want any more kids.

D. Thought six were enough and now you were going to have seven?

P. My husband told me that I wouldn't have to have any more and that I could put me on birth-control pills; and she was born in 1968, and I think I was on the pill for about three or two years, and it got where every month when I would start my period, I would just go constantly, all the time//

D. //Okay//

P. //And then when I went to the doctor, he told me that I had a spot, and they didn't know what it was. The doctor thought it was cancer, but it wasn't.

D. What was it on?

P. I think it was on my uterus.

D. Did he see the spot? Is that what was//

P. //Well, when I went to take my Pap smear, then he recommended me to another doctor, and I went to one doctor and another doctor.

D. Okay, okay, so he looked up inside you with a speculum and saw this spot.

P. Yeah, he told me then that I had to have surgery because if I didn't it could be very dangerous; and he was afraid I would get pregnant again and wouldn't be able to carry another.

The first thing that strikes me about this exchange is the way the doctor refers to the patient. After our little talk in the hall, she is transformed again, this time from *Miss* to *Mrs.* But it soon becomes clear that this change in title does not change the way the doctor positions her or the social/ideological work this positioning does. He consistently reinforces the view that any sexual expression is inappropriate for a woman whose husband has only recently died and who is not now married.

Next, I am impressed by the way the question about her earlier surgery provides interesting information and an equally interesting view of the ways the social penetrates a presumably medical discourse and does so differently for doctor and patient. The doctor asks a medical question about why the uterus was removed; and Muriel provides a medical response, excessive menstrual bleeding. Once again he challenges her. By asking how long the bleeding lasted, he checks to see that it was really excessive. As she has before, Muriel displays herself as neither overly emotional nor an incompetent reporter of her medical history. She tells him that it lasted all month. While the topic here is a medical one—excessive bleeding—doctor and patient struggle in a social/ideological register. For the doctor the social/ideological is closely tied to the medical. Satisfied that her response is reliable, he sums up: "Okay, so you had a period of time where you were bleeding for up to a month," and in the back channel the patient confirms with an "um hum." He continues, "And that's why they took your uterus out."

But for Muriel this summary does not tell the whole story. For her the medical story is embedded in the social/biographical context of her life. She takes the conversational floor and begins to provide the missing social context. She explains that after six children her husband told her that she would not have to have any more and gave her permission to take the birth-control pill. She conceived while on the pill and describes herself as upset about it. The doctor sarcastically trivializes her response by implying that her discomfort was long overdue—"Thought six were enough and now you were going to have seven?"—and, in so doing, he recirculates classic assumptions about the careless way poor women manage, or fail to manage, their fertility.

Muriel neither resists nor responds; instead she continues her narrative as if he had not spoken. While she was on the pill and after she gave birth to her last child, excessive bleeding became a problem. The doctor interrupts her story by saying, "okay," which signals that, for him, the social/biographical information being provided is extraneous. He is ready to move on. Muriel clearly does not agree. She interrupts more than once and continues answering the doctor's original question by explaining that when she started bleeding heavily, her doctor saw a spot, thought it might be cancer, and referred her to another doctor, perhaps a specialist.

Here the dreaded word, cancer, has finally been said aloud. But Muriel, not Doctor Johnson, brings it into the discussion. Once again speaking in a social/ideological register, the doctor checks Muriel's medical competence and does so without referring to cancer. He says, "So he looked up inside you . . . and saw this spot." In response, Muriel again demonstrates her competence as she tells him that her uterus was removed because "it [presumably the spot that might indicate cancer] could be very dangerous; and he [the doctor] was afraid I would get pregnant again and wouldn't be able to carry another."

While both doctor and patient are talking about a medical topic, they are doing so differently. The doctor asks medical questions and seems to want only medical responses. Although he imports social/ideological information about Muriel's reproductive competence and her competence as a patient into this medical discussion, he tries to redirect the patient from the social/biographical context of her life back to the medical topics he considers more relevant. Muriel resists. She responds to medical questions with social/biographical information about her reproductive history. In so doing she too speaks a social/ideological discourse. She links the removal of her uterus to reproductive control and reproductive control to excessive bleeding. And then she shifts the burden of responsibility to her husband and her former doctor. After six children, *her husband* told her that she would not have to have any more. *Her husband* told her she could go on the birth-control pill. *The doctor* found the spot. *The doctor* thought it might be dangerous and so her uterus was removed.

In her account, both her husband and the doctor speak for her. Her husband says no more children, and the doctor thinks the spot is dangerous but not because it might indicate cancer. It is dangerous because she might "get pregnant again and wouldn't be able to carry another."

There is a struggle over what constitutes the social here. For Muriel medical facts make sense only in the context of her everyday life. Yet, although the doctor wants just the medical facts, his medical talk is laden with social assumptions—ideological assumptions about her competence as a patient and as a woman who has failed to control her fertility. In this series of exchanges, although the patient does not explicitly challenge the doctor's ideological depiction of her and she does provide the medical facts he has asked, a struggle nevertheless ensues in a social/ideological register. Muriel does not respond to medical questions without locating them in the social/ biographical context of her life and in a social/ideological discourse that positions her as a good woman.

There are potential medical and social/ideological implications in this struggle between doctor and patient over what information is relevant. Medically, the doctor has information that the patient has had a spot that while not cancerous may well have been a precancerous lesion. If this were the case, the simple Pap smear he performed might not be adequate. The patient might be better served by a referral to an oncologist (cancer specialist) for more specific tests. No such referral is made. He also now knows that the patient, once threatened by the possibility of having cancer, may be worried about it again. This information provides the opportunity to reassure her, and a little later in the encounter he does so.

But perhaps most interesting are the struggles over competing discourses that occur in a social/ideological register. For Muriel, providing the medical facts does not tell the whole story. By immersing the facts in the social/biographical context of her life, she offers an alternative definition of both the facts and the provider-patient relationship. This definition resists the asymmetry of the medical relationship and the assumption that by virtue of her class and gender she is not able to understand what is medically relevant to the doctor.

However, although Muriel manages to squeeze social/biographical information into the medical discussion, her resistance is severely limited. Doctor Johnson has obtained a medical explanation for her prior treatment, and he clings to it while treating the social/biographical information she provides as extraneous. Therefore, neither her challenge to the asymmetry so characteristic in medical encounters nor her attempt to present herself as competent prevails. Moreover, her resistance, brief as it is, rests on her attempts to reposition herself in a social/ideological discourse, and this attempt is not without costs.

Muriel's account uses the voices of her husband and her former doctor to express her concerns. Here, men, whether doctors or husbands, know what is best for women. This presentation works well for her. If her husband's and the doctor's interests and hers overlap, she can present herself as a good woman and protect herself from the decision not to have more children and to have her uterus removed. But this protection is costly. She describes a medical relationship with a dominant doctor and a subordinate patient and a nuclear family with a dominant husband and a compliant wife. She presents herself as a woman who through no fault of her own had to stop having children; a hysterectomy was a medical necessity. While this narrative works well in protecting Muriel's identity as a good woman, a good wife, and a good patient, it also reinscribes dominant cultural assumptions about the medical relationship, the nuclear family, and women's place in both.

As if going down a checklist from our earlier conversation, the doctor continues.

> *D.* The other thing I need to know, now you told me your husband died two years ago//
>
> *P.* //My Daddy;[5] my husband will be dead twenty months tomorrow.
>
> *D.* Un huh. Have you been, excuse me, active sexually since then?
>
> *P.* Not necessarily, I mean sometimes but not like I was when we was married.
>
> *D.* Uh huh, ah, one man, different men?
>
> *P.* No just one.
>
> *D.* Okay, have you noticed any connection between when

you spot blood on your panties and having had sexual
intercourse?

   P. No.

Doctor Johnson begins this sequence by saying that there is
something he needs to know. He then moves to check the facts that
Muriel provided earlier. He asks, "Now you told me your husband
died two years ago," and the patient interrupts to tell him that it was
her Daddy that died two years ago. Her husband will be dead
"twenty months tomorrow." Once again the doctor barely pays attention to this social/biographical information. After a token ac-
knowledgment, he continues by seeking the medical information he
is really after. He hems and haws and then asks, "Have you been,
excuse me, active sexually since then?"

   The doctor's hesitancy and his "excuse me" clearly signal his discomfort discussing sexual behavior with a recently widowed, older
woman. Starting this discussion with a question about when Muriel's husband died, hemming and hawing, and asking to be excused
for inquiring about her current sexual activity import social/ideo-
logical assumptions into what is presumably a medical discussion.
The ideological message is that Muriel should be offended by such
questions—offended because such activity is inappropriate so close
to her husband's death, especially for a woman her age. This message carries cultural baggage—social/ideological baggage that reinscribes dominant assumptions about women, age, sexuality, and the
nuclear family.

   Muriel's response resists the doctor's definition of the situation
by speaking an alternative discourse about women and sexuality.
While at first glance Muriel's response may be confusing, she does
not seem to have any difficulty with the topic. She starts by saying,
"Not necessarily," but then she goes on to explain. "I mean sometimes but not like I was when we was married." From this explanation it seems clear that she and Doctor Johnson are measuring
sexual behavior differently. For the doctor the standard is an abstract normative or moral one. For Muriel it is more concrete and
tied more specifically to the context of her life. She measures her
current sexual activity against her marriage. By that standard she
has "not necessarily" been sexually active, certainly not as active as
she was when her husband was still alive.

This is an interesting set of exchanges. Although Doctor Johnson's questions are medically relevant, they are not ideologically neutral. Social/ideological assumptions clearly penetrate this discussion. Yet, as with the medical topics discussed earlier, the doctor seems to expect straightforward responses. Muriel provides such a response to the first question. Her husband "will be dead twenty months tomorrow." However, because she and Doctor Johnson are using different social criteria, her response to the second question is quite different. Rather than just providing the medically relevant information requested, she embeds her answer in the social/biographical context of her life, and a double struggle ensues.

Here, we see doctor and patient simultaneously struggling over what constitutes a legitimate medical explanation and what constitutes appropriate sexual behavior for women. Although Muriel responds to the question about whether she is sexually active, she resists both the doctor's definition of the situation, in which the social/biographical context of her life is not a relevant topic for discussion, and his ideological message that there is something wrong with her or that her behavior is somehow inappropriate. Muriel speaks about her current sexual behavior as if the only problem it presents is that it does not occur with the same frequency as it did when she was married. In so doing she positions herself as a good woman even if recently widowed and sexually active. But while she resists, there is no evidence that she prevails.

Although Muriel provides information from the social/biographical context of her life that may be relevant to Doctor Johnson's diagnosis and treatment, he does not pick up her cues. Muriel has consistently referred to stress in her life. She has told the doctor that her father and her husband died within four months of each other, and that while sexually active, she is not as active as she once had been. The doctor does not ask whether either the deaths or the change in her sexual activity has been a problem for her. In other words, he does not incorporate the social/biographical information she has struggled to provide into the medical discussion.

Muriel's social/ideological presentation of herself as a sexual woman is similarly ineffective. Doctor Johnson's next question clearly indicates that despite Muriel's resistance, his conception of her has not changed at all. He asks whether Muriel has had sex with one man or with different men. While we cannot be certain that

Muriel hears the ideological message implied here, we can be sure that she does not respond to it. She gives a straightforward response, "No, just one," as if responding to a medical question.

Again, this is an interesting exchange. The doctor's question may be soliciting necessary medical information, but it also reinscribes the hegemonic assumptions that Muriel and Doctor Johnson have been struggling over. While Doctor Johnson and Muriel are both Appalachian, Doctor Johnson recirculates the dominant views of this community, and Muriel does not. The ideological assumptions about women and sexuality that the doctor has expressed, and Muriel has resisted, are all too common in the Southeast, a part of the United States often referred to as the Bible Belt. These assumptions are based on religious beliefs that legitimate a woman's sexuality only for reproduction and in the confines of the family. Perhaps this symmetry between Doctor Johnson's views and the dominant views of the community undermines Muriel's resistance. But if so, this symmetry is not without medical and social/ideological costs, which are clearly in evidence in Doctor Johnson's silence as well as in his question.

He does not reassure Muriel that being sexually active is a normal part of life or that her medical problem is not retribution for her immorality. Given his membership in the fundamentalist religious culture of the Appalachian region, perhaps it is unreasonable to expect him to. This membership is also in evidence in his question, which implies that a good woman would not be sexually active outside of marriage and certainly not with more than one man.

But perhaps even more striking are the ways these cultural assumptions are visible in Doctor Johnson's clinical practice.

He initiates the topic of sex and solicits information about the patient's sexual history, albeit with coaching from me. But while this information has clinical significance, he does not follow through. He now knows that even though Muriel's husband has been dead less than two years, she is sexually active—information that is relevant for his diagnosis. A differential diagnosis for a woman with vaginal bleeding seven years after a hysterectomy should include sexually transmitted diseases. But to test for sexually transmitted diseases is to acknowledge Muriel's sexuality in ways that are at odds with the doctor's normative frame of reference. By not testing, he keeps his social/ideological definition of the situation firmly in place.

Muriel's responses are equally complex. Although Doctor Johnson solicits specific information abstracted from the social/biographical context of her life, Muriel does not always provide it that way. Similarly, even though the doctor has evidenced his discomfort with treating Muriel as a sexually active woman, Muriel does not just passively accept this social/ideological definition. On some occasions she provides the information requested in a straightforward manner. But other times she refuses to put the context of her life aside or to accept the doctor's definition of her.

This interaction provides a particularly clear example of the ways social/ideological assumptions influence what purports to be objective medical treatment. While Muriel's resistance provokes a struggle over competing discourses about the nature of the medical relationship and about women and sexuality, she does not prevail. The doctor's ideological assumptions continue to shape his behavior. Through this behavior, he revivifies his position as the dominant interactional partner, the one who defines legitimate and illegitimate topics for discussion, and he delivers care in ways that reproduce his cultural understanding of women and sexuality.

My conversation with Doctor Johnson in the hall is strongly in evidence in the next set of exchanges as well.

> D. All right, Miss Whales, let me tell you what I think, okay? When you came, when you first, when I first started talking to you today, I was worried, all right. When a lady comes in and sits down and starts talking about vaginal bleeding, the first thing anybody thinks about . . . what did you think about?
> P. Well, I didn't really know.
> D. Well, ah, what did you think about though? What were you really worried about?
> P. I was more or less worried about, maybe, that I would have cancer.
> D. And that's what I was talking about. All right, so that's the first thing we have to decide, whether or not this bleeding is from some sort of tumor or growth or something. I don't

think it is. I don't see any indication that you have any growths within your vagina, okay. (P. Okay.) I do see indication that you have an infection, probably two infections. One of them is called trichomoniasis, and that's a fancy name for an amoeba, a little one-cell animal if you will, that might spread in moist, dark, warm places, and the female vagina is one such place. You can get trichomoniasis in a number of ways. You can get it swimming in lakes and streams. You can get it through sexual intercourse. But I'm just telling you that that's just one of the ways you can get it. You also have nonspecific vaginitis, if you want to call it that, which needs to be treated. Luckily, both the things we need to treat can be treated with the same medicine. You only have to take one medicine, okay? The other thing is whether or not we need to treat your boyfriend, the man you have sexual intercourse with. I think he might also have trichomoniasis. Is he still in this area?

P. Um hm.

D. Okay, uh, you can do it one of two ways. We can have him come in and see me, have him see another doctor, or we can, the worse way to do it is to give you some medicine and have him take it. (P. Okay.) Okay, because medically, legally that's a little hairy situation, me giving you medicine to give him; and I've never seen him and I don't know what he is allergic to or what he is doing or in fact if he even has this infection. Okay, although men can get it, that doesn't mean that he necessarily, that he has it. What do you want to do?

P. Well, that's a tough situation; that's a tough answer.

D. A tough situation it sure is.

P. Um, I don't have no choice, do I?

D. Well, if he does have trich and he has sexual intercourse with someone else, he can give it to them. If he has sexual intercourse with you again, he can give it right back to you. I think he needs to be treated, okay?

P. Okay.

D. If you want to have him come and see me, I'll examine him and treat him for it, okay? If you want to have him go to his doctor, then his doctor can call and talk to me about it, all right? We're not talking about VD or anything like that.

We're talking about an organism that is transmitted vaginally. Okay, that doesn't say that you got this venereal. But you could have given it to him, or he could have given it to you, or you could have gotten it in a lake or a river or in a public bathroom, okay?

P. Yeah, 'cause I only went swimming one time this whole year.

D. Do you drink alcohol?

P. Yes, occasionally.

D. I don't want you to drink any alcohol as long as you are taking this medication, okay?

P. Okay.

By the way this exchange starts, it seems that the doctor is going to bring cancer into the discussion and reassure Muriel about her probable concerns. But after starting with "let me tell you what I think," he pauses and asks her what she thinks about her vaginal bleeding and whether she is really worried. When Muriel responds by saying, "Well, I didn't really know," he asks again. Finally, the patient, not the doctor, once again speaks the unspeakable word, cancer, and states that she is "more or less worried" that she has cancer.

Once she mentions cancer, Doctor Johnson begins what I assume he intends as reassurance. He reveals that the medical task is to decide whether the bleeding is related to "some sort of tumor or growth." He then tells her that although he sees no indication of "any growths," he has seen evidence of two infections—trichomoniasis and vaginitis—both of which can be contracted in a variety of ways. He names swimming and sexual intercourse as two possible sources of contagion and informs her that, however contracted, both infections need to be treated. He explains they can be treated with the same "medicine." He then raises an issue that never gets resolved: whether to treat her boyfriend. While on the surface this is clearly medical talk about a medical problem, there is a social/ideological subtext. The topics that the doctor does not address without prompting from me—cancer and sexuality—carry a social charge that seems to have real consequences. While the doctor inquires about why Muriel had a hysterectomy, he seems much less comfortable exploring her potential fears about cancer. He seems unable to even speak the word, and when, after his prompting, Muriel does so, his reassurance is brief. "I don't see any indication that you have growths in your vagina."

The problems Muriel's sexuality raise for him are both much more complex and, at first glance, not as visible. Doctor Johnson opens this exchange by referring to Muriel again as Miss Whales. He then tells her that neither trichomoniasis nor vaginitis is a venereal disease. He explains that the infections she has may be transmitted through sexual intercourse, through swimming in lakes and streams, or from public bathrooms. Although he does not ask her how she thinks she was infected, he does inform her that her sexual partner also may have trichomoniasis and needs to be treated. He suggests two (but he presents three) ways the "boyfriend" can be treated: Doctor Johnson or another doctor in the clinic can treat him; he can go to his own doctor, who can call Doctor Johnson; or Doctor Johnson, despite the medical and legal risks, can prescribe medication for Muriel to share with him.

Although this seems like a perfectly reasonable discussion of the medical facts, it is shot through with social/ideological assumptions. Doctor Johnson again sends the message that as an older, recently widowed woman Muriel does not conform to dominant cultural assumptions about women and sexuality. By saying "your boyfriend," then correcting himself and calling him the man Muriel has sex with (without establishing which he is), and finally asking whether he is *still* in the area, the doctor implies that Muriel is engaging in casual, perhaps even promiscuous, sex. When the doctor explains the need for treating her partner by talking about how the infection can be transmitted to other sexual partners, this message continues. Perhaps Muriel and her partner are engaging in sexual intercourse with each other and with other people. Perhaps for both Muriel and her partner their sexual relations are no more than casual sex with a transient partner. Or perhaps she is having sexual intercourse with only one regular partner, and he is her boyfriend, but he is sexually active with more than one woman. Whichever fantasy you prefer, the message seems to be that if "Miss Whales" is sexually active outside of marriage and so soon after her husband's death, she is not a good woman.

Even though these messages are not stated in so many words,

Muriel's responses imply that she has heard and understood them. After the doctor suggests that either partner could have given the infections to the other or that they could have gotten them through swimming or public bathrooms, Muriel responds, "I only went swimming one time this whole year." While she has easily admitted being sexually active even as a recent widow, she struggles here to avoid the stigma associated with sexually transmitted infections.

Despite cultural myths to the contrary, Muriel seems to recognize that the most frequent source of transmission is sexual intercourse with infected partners, not lakes or public bathrooms. Nevertheless, by accepting the myth, she can reposition herself. Her luck may be bad—she went swimming only once and she got an infection—but she salvages her morality. To reclaim her identity, Muriel gives up her definition of the situation. No longer is she a good woman even if recently widowed and sexually active. In the face of a sexually transmitted disease she repositions herself in ways that not only replay the good woman/bad woman duality but recirculate the very messages she has been resisting. She is a good woman because she did not contract these infections through sexual intercourse. She became infected while swimming.

Reclaiming her identity as a good woman by not resisting the doctor's messages about women and sexuality has additional medical costs, which include inadequate medical care and the risk of a recurring infection. Doctor Johnson is consistent. He has difficulty with Muriel's sexual behavior. This difficulty is reflected both in what he says and does and in what he leaves unsaid and undone. For example, even though he finds that Muriel has two infections that are vaginally transmitted, Doctor Johnson does not screen her for other, potentially more serious venereal diseases.[6] And even though he says, "We're not talking about VD or anything like that," he does not make a clear distinction between an infection that is vaginally transmitted and a venereal disease.

Each lack of follow-up reflects his social/ideological assumptions, and each affects his clinical practice. Perhaps this effect emerges most clearly in the discussion about treating Muriel's boyfriend. After presenting the available treatment options, Doctor Johnson asks Muriel what she wants to do. Her response is telling. She says, "Well that's a tough situation; that's a tough answer," and concludes by saying, "Um, I don't have no choice, do I?" It seems clear that Muriel cannot differentiate between a vaginally transmitted infection and a venereal disease. What's tough is that, given her lack of clarity, she is not eager to go home and tell her boyfriend that medicine has been prescribed for an infection and he has to take it too. She does not want him to think she has a venereal disease or to accuse him of having one that he passed on to her.

While I would be the first to agree that patients be given the facts and encouraged to make their own medical decisions, the doctor does not pick up Muriel's cues and inquire about her perceptions or feelings. Why is the situation tough? What are the potential consequences for her of having "no choice"? Does she have enough information to explain to her boyfriend the difference between a venereal disease and a vaginally transmitted infection? How does she feel about telling her man friend that she has a vaginal infection and that he needs to be checked by a doctor? How does she think her boyfriend will respond? Does she feel in danger? Is she afraid that her boyfriend will think that she has been sexually promiscuous and leave her? Might he think that she has been unfaithful and beat her? The doctor does not ask these or related social/biographical questions. Neither does he push for a medical decision, and the patient does not make one. She leaves the clinic without a prescription for her sexual partner and without making an appointment for him to come in to be checked.

Although Muriel has not prevailed, she has struggled valiantly against the doctor's social/ideological definition of the situation. But while it was one thing for her to bring the social/biographical context of her life into the discussion, to defend her competence, or to guard her identity as a sexually active woman even though older and recently widowed, it is quite another to protect herself against the stigma associated with a venereal disease. On this topic there seems to be no conflicting position for her, no oppositional discourse that she can circulate. But when she gives up this battle, the way is left open for Doctor Johnson's cultural assumptions to structure his clinical practice, and they do. Even though the consequence is inadequate medical care, Muriel does not resist, and we would not expect her to. Most patients do not have access to the kind of medical information that would provide a basis for resistance of this kind.

The medical encounter concludes with Doctor Johnson explaining how the patient should take her medicine and setting the stage for her to return.

> *D.* You have to take one tablet three times a day for seven days. Okay? If you start, after you finish this, if you start having vaginal bleeding, I want to see you then, when it happens, when it's going on, and not a week later. Okay? So if you notice any vaginal bleeding, you call my girls and say, "Hey, I'm bleeding, and he said when I'm bleeding, I need to come in." All right. If that Pap smear I took comes back normal, I'm going to call you and say that your Pap smear is normal. If it is abnormal, I won't call you. All right// (P.// All right.), and we'll get this all straightened out. I want you to come back in a couple, three or four weeks, whatever, and we can talk some more about the things that are bothering you. All right//
>
> *P.//* Well, a lot of things bother me here lately, 'cause I know I'm real upset, very much; and I know I sit and cry a lot, and I know that's not right, but I don't know what I'm going to do about it.
>
> *D.* You got to where you don't care what your house looks like?
>
> *P.* I got to where I'm real particular about my house. I know that I always want to keep it clean . . .

In this closing section of the medical encounter Doctor Johnson sums up medically. He tells Muriel how to take her medicine and establishes that vaginal bleeding is a medically significant symptom that necessitates medical attention. If, after she finishes taking her medicine, she has another episode of bleeding, he wants to see her. He also reaffirms the importance of seeing Muriel again by telling her how to subvert the bureaucratic organization of the practice. "If you notice any vaginal bleeding, you call my girls and say, 'Hey, I'm bleeding, and he said when I'm bleeding, I need to come in.'"

Putting aside my discomfort with his use of "girls" to refer to the secretary and the nurse who work with him, the doctor certainly establishes vaginal bleeding as a legitimate reason for seeking medical attention, and, thereby, for the first and only time in this encounter, he affirms Muriel's competence as a patient.

While still speaking in a medical voice, he is much less clear about the results of the Pap smear. The doctor tells Muriel that if the Pap smear is normal, he will call and tell her so, but if it is abnormal, he will not. Patients are usually told just the opposite. It is hard to imagine why he set things up this way. What is the patient to do if she does not hear from him? How long should she wait and worry?

Without any further explanation, he moves from medical to social/biographical topics, saying that he wants the patient to return at some loosely specified future time to talk some more about the things that are bothering her. He raises here the very issues she has repeatedly and unsuccessfully tried to talk about in this encounter. The doctor brings the topic of the patient's life into the discussion, and Muriel responds in kind. She affirms that there are lots of things bothering her, that she know she is very upset—so upset that she cries a lot. She tells him that she knows this is not right, but she does not know what she is going to do about it.

At first glance the doctor's response to Muriel's trouble telling seems incongruous. Muriel has just described how upset she is, and Doctor Johnson asks her whether she has "got to where you don't care what your house looks like." But if this talk about the social/biographical context of Muriel's life is filtered through a medical frame, it is not incongruous at all. The talk about the troubles in Muriel's life have potential medical ramifications, and Doctor Johnson responds to one of these ramifications.[7] He seems to hear that the "things" bothering Muriel may be serious. She may be describing a clinical depression, and this kind of depression needs medical treatment.

This hearing is reflected in his question about housekeeping—a question with clear social/ideological overtones. It is medically well documented that depression interferes with people's ability to perform—their ability to live their lives and do their jobs. Doctor Johnson is inquiring about Muriel's ability to do her job, her ability to keep her house clean. His normative assumption that housekeeping is women's work is reflected in his question and in Muriel's response. Muriel presents herself as mentally healthy, saying, "I got to where I'm real particular about my house. I know that I always want to keep it clean." In accepting the doctor's social/ideological definition of the situation, she may have saved herself from the shame of mental illness, but there are costs. She participates in recirculating hegemonic assumptions about women's domestic responsibilities, and as the closing moments of the encounter demonstrate, she frees the doctor from any further consideration of the troubles in her life.

As the encounter is ending, Muriel tries once again to enumerate the problems in her life. She talks about how hard it is to keep the house clean with so many people living in a trailer. She brings up arguments among her children and how hard they are to deal with in the context of her recent losses of her Daddy and her husband. But since Muriel keeps her house clean, her complaints do not indicate a clinical depression and, therefore, do not need medical treatment.

Doctor Johnson consistently opts for a narrow medical definition of the situation that separates genuine medical business from extraneous social/biographical talk. For Muriel, the social/biographical provides the context in which to make sense of the medical. While she tries repeatedly to discuss the social context of her life, she is not successful. The social topics Muriel tries to raise seem to be of interest to the doctor only if they have medical consequences. This definition of the situation not only affects the way care is provided but also influences Muriel's willingness to return. While Doctor Johnson suggests that Muriel make another appointment to discuss the things that have been bothering her, she does not. If she has not been successful on this visit, when she had a legitimate medical problem, why would she be successful on subsequent visits? Furthermore, as a poor woman how could she justify another trip to the doctor? In the three years that I followed her records, neither she nor her man friend came to the clinic.

Although Doctor Johnson separates the medical and the social/biographical, he simultaneously transports social/ideological assumptions into presumably medical discussions, and in this social/ideological register doctor and patient struggle. Muriel resists Doctor Johnson's repeated depiction of her as less than competent—

a description with clear class and gender implications. She also resists his insistence on dominant cultural notions about women and sexuality. With her resistance she circulates an alternative discourse—a discourse in which women are competent to talk about their medical histories and in which it is perfectly normal for older, recently widowed women to be sexually active. And in so doing she challenges hegemonic assumptions about women as well as the asymmetry of the medical relationship and their respective positions in it.

But Muriel does not prevail. Whether Doctor Johnson's definition of the situation is medical or social/ideological, he persistently circulates dominant discourses that position him as the medical expert and Muriel as a poor, incompetent, lower-class woman with loose sexual morals. And notwithstanding Muriel's resistance, his definition of the situation consistently succeeds. While Muriel resists repeatedly, her position is not as consistent. On three occasions she participates in recirculating the dominant understandings she has been struggling against. When she protects her identity from the stigma of choosing to have no more children by placing the decision-making capacity with her husband and her doctor, she recirculates hegemonic understandings about domestic and medical relationships. Similarly when she protects her identity from the stigma of a venereal disease, she participates in the reproduction of dominant understandings about women and sexuality. And when she defends herself against the shame associated with being a poor housekeeper, she reinscribes hegemonic notions about women's proper role in the home.

It is not, then, that doctor and patient each speak a single discourse and through these discourses compete to define the situations being discussed. Rather we see here two struggles. In the first the patient tries unsuccessfully to insert social/biographical information into a discourse defined as medical by the doctor. However, the doctor both raises the topic of the patient's life and inserts a social/ideological discourse into the discussions. The second is a struggle between competing social/ideological discourses both within the patient and between the patient and the doctor. While the patient is sometimes ambivalent, the doctor is not. Whether discussing social/ideological or medical topics, he pushes to control the definition of the situation, and he consistently succeeds. But his success carries high costs. It influences the way he practices medicine, shaping both the delivery of health care and the reasons for the patient's noncompliance. And, in the end, with Muriel's help or without it, hegemonic assumptions are revivified. In this process dominant understandings about the status of doctor and patient, man and woman are reproduced.

SIX

COMPLAINTS CODED AS MEDICAL
The Nursing Consultation

In this encounter the nurse practitioner, Claudia Sussen, and the patient, Pat Scott, are not meeting each other for the first time. This is not an initial visit for an urgent problem. It is a routine visit for a chronic medical condition—diabetes. The medical consultation opens with Claudia walking into the examining room where Pat Scott sits waiting in one of the two available chairs. She is a slim, neatly dressed, well-groomed fifty-four-year-old black woman who hardly looks her age. Claudia greets her, takes the other chair, and opens the encounter by picking up the thread of prior discussions and checking on the status of ongoing medical problems.

> *N.P.* How are you?
> *P.* I'm good.
> *N.P.* Haven't seen you for a while.
> *P.* Yeah.
> *N.P.* That's good.
> *P.* Yeah.
> *N.P.* I guess it means you're okay?
> *P.* Yeah, well, so far.
> *N.P.* I see that you came in and saw the dermatologist for your foot. (P. Yeah.) How is it?
> *P.* It's good.
> *N.P.* When are you supposed to come back for that?
> *P.* In, ah, three months.
> *N.P.* Are you using the medicine?

P. Yes.

N.P. You're just cutting away a little bit of it.

P. I still can't do those (unintelligible), go down too far, and it starts bleeding.

N.P. Is it better?

P. Oh, yes, it's much better. I can walk on it good, . . . as long as I keep that hard piece out of it, I can go for days without it bothering me.

N.P. Good. Tell me what medicine you're taking now.

P. (A slight shrug but no response.)

N.P. What do you think you take? You take a pill for your sugar?

P. Yeah.

N.P. How often?

P. Um, once a day.

N.P. Okay, just want to check. You did fine. You got it.

From the onset this interaction looks different from many, if not most, medical encounters. It certainly begins differently from Muriel's encounter with Doctor Johnson. The patient waits for the provider sitting in a chair dressed, not sitting on the examining table undressed. When Claudia enters the examining room, she greets Pat, takes the chair opposite her, and opens the interview by commenting that she has not seen her for a while. Both the spatial positioning and the way provider and patient greet each other speak to a kind of symmetry not usually in evidence in medical encounters. But they also suggest a kind of tension not in evidence in the medical consultation—a tension also visible in the nurse practitioner–patient encounter discussed in Chapter Four. As in most provider-patient encounters, the nurse practitioner is interactionally dominant. This dominance is reflected in the ways she initiates the encounter and the topics to be discussed, and it becomes clearer as the consultation unfolds. However, there is also a kind of symmetry not usually in evidence in medical encounters—a symmetry represented in these opening moments by the way nurse practitioner and patient relate to each other verbally and nonverbally. The tension, then, is between the symmetry of what Davis (1988) refers to as a "friendship frame" and the more typical asymmetry of a medical consultation.

In addition, the difference between an initial visit for an urgent problem and a routine visit for a chronic problem is immediately apparent. There is no presenting complaint to be elicited. Instead, as a primary-care provider, the nurse practitioner picks up the threads of prior medical discussions. Claudia asks Pat how she is and comments that she has not seen her for a while, so she must be okay. Pat affirms that she is doing well but, by saying, "Yeah, well, so far," signals some concern, which Claudia does not address. Instead she continues by checking about the patient's foot problem. Has she seen the dermatologist who rotates through the clinic, is she using the medicine prescribed, when is she to go to that doctor again, and does her foot feel better?

The contrast with the medical encounter between Doctor Johnson and Muriel, discussed in the previous chapter, is particularly interesting. Unlike the doctor, the nurse practitioner does not seem to be using these questions as an opportunity to challenge Pat's competence as a patient. This stance is particularly striking in light of a cultural mythology that suggests that poor African American women are anything but competent. Instead, Claudia accepts Pat's responses unproblematically. She suggests that if the patient has not been in to see her, she must have been feeling all right. She checks on a referral she made and ascertains that it has been helpful.

In these interactions the nurse practitioner is coordinating Pat's health care while also performing more subtle social/ideological work. Status differentiations are minimized as the identities of nurse practitioner and patient are negotiated. Claudia is providing an alternative discourse, one that neither reinscribes dominant cultural assumptions about poor African American women nor simply recirculates the asymmetry so characteristic of the medical relationship. Even though Claudia does not bring the full force of her professional status to bear, this status provides a site from which to reinforce her professional dominance or to undermine it. And in this interaction she does both.

Claudia's support of Pat as a competent patient is probably clearest in the discussion about medication. She asks what medicine Pat is taking, and Pat shrugs and does not reply. Her shrug and her silence could easily be taken as ignorance, and that ignorance could just as easily be attributed to her race, gender, or class. The nurse practitioner does not make this assumption. Instead she reframes her questions and encourages the patient to respond, encourages her to demonstrate her competence. "You take a pill for your sugar?" "How often?" When the patient responds, Claudia says, "Okay, just wanted to check. You did fine. You got it."

While discussing medical topics, Claudia has been offering an alternative discourse; however, the admission "just wanted to check" and the evaluation "You did fine. You got it" reinscribe the status of the nurse practitioner as medical expert and a view of Pat as a less than competent and reliable adult. Although it may be good clinical practice to check that a patient is taking medicine properly, the way this check is made here does ideological work. Perhaps this difference is easiest to see by comparison. Imagine a middle-class white woman being complimented because she knows that she is taking a medication for diabetes correctly. Even more far-fetched is to imagine this kind of encounter with a middle-class white man. Parents check on children, and teachers evaluate students. For Claudia to check on and evaluate Pat's understanding in this way infantilizes her.

But perhaps most interesting is the way this shift in discursive positions is in opposition to Claudia's prior support of Pat as a competent person. While Claudia is asking medical questions and checking on the patient's health status, she is navigating between competing social/ideological discourses, making visible the tension between them. Moreover, whether she is offering an alternative to dominant cultural assumptions or recirculating these same assumptions, Pat has not resisted her definition of the situation.

Although not stated explicitly, social/ideological assumptions penetrate presumably medical discourse and simultaneously do two different kinds of ideological work. They reproduce and resist an asymmetrical medical relationship with a dominant provider and a subordinate patient as they reinscribe and undermine the kind of provider-patient relationship nurse practitioners claim to offer. And, at the same time, they produce a conception of the patient both as a competent and as a less than competent adult, resisting and recirculating an image of Pat with clear racial, class, and gender implications.

Claudia continues picking up the threads of Pat's medical history.

N.P. I want to check your blood pressure. Can you take your sweater off? Can I just take a look at that place on your arm that brought you in in the first place? Remember that sore that you had?

P. Yeah.

N.P. You still got a little thing there, don't you? Are you working on that?

P. Yeah.

N.P. With what?

P. I take that off, and I wash it. The scab comes on, and then every night a little bump comes up. I don't know why. That's a little bit of pus right there, but it doesn't bother me at all. It doesn't hurt or anything. It's got a yellow spot there. It looks like a little bit of pus.

N.P. How often do you get that scab off that?

P. Um, I got it off twice, but I had to use Vaseline to soften it up and take it off. It comes off easy.

N.P. It comes off easy?

P. Yeah.

N.P. How long did you have to keep the Vaseline on?

P. Uh, not that long.

After asking medical questions and checking on the status of Pat's health, Claudia moves to a physical examination. She tells Pat that she wants to take her blood pressure and to "take a look at that place on your arm that brought you in in the first place." Claudia is concerned about the scab because diabetics are particularly prone to infections that both are difficult to treat and can exacerbate their disease. On observation Claudia sees that the spot is still there. She questions whether Pat is working on healing it and, after Pat responds that she is, asks, "With what?" Pat describes how she washes her arm and how a scab forms. Claudia then asks her, "How often do you get that scab off?"

In this exchange Claudia is asking medical questions, and Pat is responding in kind. This questioning treats Pat as competent. However, as the exchange continues, that treatment begins to change. Pat explains that she has used Vaseline to soften the scab. Doing so makes it come off easily, and she has twice been able to remove it. The nurse practitioner makes a question of the patient's assertion that "it [the scab] comes off easy." In so doing she questions Pat's competence both to care for herself and to report accurately on the way she has done so—questions with class, gender, and racial implications. Although there is no way to know whether Pat hears this challenge, it is clear that she does not respond to it, does not resist Claudia's definition of the situation.

Claudia then begins to remove the scab herself. As she does so her behavior both challenges Pat's description and demonstrates the tensions between competing discourses—tensions that produce a struggle conducted in a medical register but with a social/ideological subtext.

> N.P. I want to see what's under there.
> P. Oh, you hurt it. You can't get it off like that.
> N.P. With water? I have Vaseline.
> P. I don't take it off with water.
> N.P. Well, the first time you came in we took it off with water. I guess it was a lot different then. It was really infected. Well, if you think Vaseline will work, we'll use Vaseline.

This is an interesting exchange. Claudia applies a little water and attempts to lift the scab. Pat, who has challenged neither the alternative production of her as a competent patient and a more or less equal interactional partner nor the more hegemonic presentation of her as a subordinate whose competence is at least questionable, resists this behavioral display.

Pat stops Claudia, saying, "Oh, you hurt it. You can't get it off like that." Claudia checks to see whether she is understanding the patient's complaint. She says, "With water? I have Vaseline." There is an implied criticism both in Pat's statement that she does not take the scab off with water and in her tone of voice. Claudia responds to this criticism by defending herself. Looking at Pat's medical records, Claudia explains that when Pat first came in the scab was removed easily with water but perhaps that was because it was "really infected" then. She then begins to remove the scab using Vaseline, and Pat says, "Yeah, Vaseline doesn't hurt." This comment can be heard as a positive evaluation.

Although Pat does not challenge the linguistic message that she may not know what she is talking about, she certainly challenges its behavioral manifestation. And she prevails. After Claudia defends herself, providing the grounds to continue to see her as both competent and humane even if mistaken, she removes the scab as Pat directed. Pat comments on this treatment by evaluating and praising Claudia's actions.

This interaction is unusual in several respects. Although unfortunately it is all too common for providers to challenge the competence of patients, it is all too rare for patients to challenge the competence of providers, especially about medical matters. If making such a challenge is unusual for most patients, it is even more unusual for lower-status patients, and, by most accoutns, as a poor, African American woman, Pat is a lower-status patient. In fact I have never seen a woman patient challenge a doctor and put him on the defensive.[1]

It is even more unusual for providers to defend themselves or to accord patients medical expertise. In my experience doctors sanction patients for trying to take control, especially in medical matters (Fisher and Groce 1990). Yet, in this instance Pat intrudes onto Claudia's medical turf, presents herself as the highest authority on her scab, and is not taken to task. Instead, her resistance is successful. She is accorded the status of medical expert. The nurse practitioner both complies with her directive about the most appropriate way to remove the scab and defends her status as a competent provider. Not only does the patient's definition of the situation prevail—a medical definition—but, in addition, she rewards Claudia for following her directions. If it is unusual to put medical providers on the defensive about medical topics, it is even more unusual for patients to evaluate them. And it is striking that instead of calling Pat to task for her inappropriate behavior, Claudia defends herself and follows Pat's directions.

We are seeing here how tensions between conflicting social/ideological discourses get worked out in concrete interactions. Provider and patient are negotiating tensions between discourses that reinscribe and those that resist both the characteristic asymmetry of the medical relationship and dominant cultural assumptions about race, class, and gender. On some occasions the nurse practitioner resists the asymmetry of the medical relationship, and on others she recirculates it. At times the patient is treated as competent, and at other times her competence is undermined. Although there are clear class, gender, and race implications when undermining occurs, the patient rarely resists.

However, as provider and patient navigate between these discursive positions, the nurse practitioner consistently is the dominant interactional partner. At one and the same time, she relies on her institutional location and distances herself from it. She sets the tone of the consultation, defines the situation, and establishes the topics for discussion. But she also provides the interactional space for Pat to challenge her competence, to evaluate her performance, and to resist and change her definition of the situation.

With the scab removed, Claudia continues to pursue medical topics and accords Pat the status of a competent patient. She checks Pat's blood pressure and questions whether she is checking her urine for sugar and how she does so. Claudia then signals a transition from a medical discussion to the social/biographical context of Pat's life by saying, "That's it."

On prior visits Pat has described herself as isolated—an isolation that may have medical implications. In the past Claudia has encouraged her to be a little more social.

> *N.P.* That's it. How are you spending your time these days?
>
> *P.* Uh, I (long pause).
>
> *N.P.* What do you do?
>
> *P.* Well, my sisters be coming over to sing.
>
> *N.P.* You weren't doing that before. What made the difference?
>
> *P.* I don't know. Maybe I just got lonesome. (Both laugh.)
>
> *N.P.* You're something else! Have you been doing that, having people over?
>
> *P.* No.
>
> *N.P.* This is the first time?
>
> *P.* Uh huh.
>
> *N.P.* What are you going to sing?
>
> *P.* I'm thinking, I don't know even what I'm going to feed them.
>
> *N.P.* What do you like?

P. For me, I like almost anything.

N.P. Uh huh.

P. I'm having two of my sisters and two ladies in the church.

N.P. Uh huh.

P. (unintelligible)

N.P. That's wonderful. Tell me how it goes, okay?

P. Okay, I will.

N.P. I think that's great. Okay.

The nurse practitioner, not the patient, opens the exchange by moving from discussions about medical topics to a discussion about Pat's social isolation. After concluding that at this time isolation is not posing a problem in Pat's life, Claudia signals her waning interest in this topic. At first the shift is subtle. Instead of the kind of strong response she has given earlier—"You're something else!"—she responds to the information the patient is providing with two minimal, token responses ("uh huh"). When Pat continues to explain how she combats social isolation, Claudia moves more overtly toward changing the topic. She affirms Pat's move toward being more social once more. In so doing, she evaluates Pat's behavior, and then, signaling a transition by saying "okay," she picks up the threads of earlier consultations and initiates another medical topic.

These topic shifts are interesting. The nurse practitioner clearly is in charge. She terminates the discussion of one topic and initiates and pursues another. As she does so she evaluates how Pat lives her life. When she has heard enough, she closes one discussion by initiating another. Here, substantively and interactionally, the nursing consultation looks much like the medical encounter discussed in the previous chapter. By evaluating the way Pat is moving to counter her social isolation, Claudia reproduces the asymmetry characteristic of the provider-patient relationship. However, there are also significant differences. Claudia directs the discussion to the social/biographical context of Pat's life—a topic all too often ignored in medical encounters (Todd 1989). When at the end of this exchange the nurse practitioner returns to a medical topic, both the form and the content of the discussion are unusual.

After summing up her medical findings, Claudia moves on to

discuss possible iatrogenic effects of Pat's blood pressure medication.

> *N.P.* I think that's great. Okay. Last time we checked your
> sugar it was good. You're taking the same medication you
> were taking. Your blood pressure's doing well. One of the
> things with this blood pressure medicine, sometimes it does,
> it causes people to be a little bit depressed. Have you noticed
> being down or sad?
> *P.* I don't know if it's the medicine. I can't blame it on the
> medicine 'cause sometimes I get depressed, sometimes,
> anyway even before . . .

And a little later:

> *N.P.* Okay. What do you do when you're depressed?
> *P.* Get up and try to do something.
> *N.P.* So it's not a big problem in your life at this point?
> *P.* Uh huh.

Claudia begins this exchange by sharing information about Pat's chronic health problems. Pat is a diabetic, and she has high blood pressure. Claudia assures her that both conditions are under control.

While speaking in the voice of medicine, Claudia is speaking an alternative discourse that does social/ideological work. By sharing medical information, she positions Pat as a competent patient, minimizes the distance between provider and patient, and undermines the characteristic asymmetry in the medical relationship. In so doing she simultaneously resists dominant cultural assumptions about poor African American women. If this is unusual behavior for a medical provider, and in my experience it is, it is even more unusual for providers to link medical discussions to the social/biographical context of patients' lives. And this is just what Claudia does. The next topic she raises is the iatrogenic potential of a prescribed medication Pat routinely takes.

It is well known that medication for high blood pressure often has adverse side effects and that depression is a commonly associated effect. Unfortunately, providers often fail to inform patients of this potential or to initiate a discussion about iatrogenic consequences like depressions. Instead, they commonly assume that if you tell patients that a medication might have a side effect or if you inquire about that side effect, you induce the undesired effect. The implication is that patients are suggestible and that iatrogenicity is, at least in part, a matter of mind over body.

Claudia does the unusual by mentioning the iatrogenic consequence of a prescribed medication, especially in the absence of a strong cue from the patient and especially because that consequence is a mental state. She says, "One of the things with this blood-pressure medicine, sometimes it does, it causes people to be a little depressed." She then asks whether Pat has "noticed being down or sad." Although the question could open a Pandora's box, Pat does not respond in the way traditional expectations suggest. She acknowledges getting depressed sometimes, but she neither floods the interaction with a barrage of social/biographical talk nor blames the medication for the troubles in her life. In fact Pat, not the nurse practitioner, argues that whatever depression she has experienced cannot be linked conclusively to her medication.

Having opened the door to the social/biographical context of Pat's life, Claudia picks up her cue and inquires about depression. In most medical encounters this kind of social/biographical information and this kind of talk about the patient's mental state are bypassed in favor of medical topics.[2] After concluding that at this time depression is not a big problem in Pat's life, Claudia once again initiates a new topic—preventive care. Although this is a medical topic, it is also frequently left uncovered in medical encounters.

It seems that the nurse practitioner as primary-care provider has covered all the bases—medical and social/biographical. But, in doing so, she has neither abandoned the authority usually associated with the provider-patient relationship nor spoken in the neutral voice of medical science. Claudia both invokes and distances herself from the authority associated with her professional status. And her talk, whether medical or social/biographical, is as ideologically saturated as the other providers' has been. As she moves on to discuss preventive health measures and to do some patient education, these facets of the consultation emerge clearly.

N.P. You have not had a Pap smear here.

P. What's that?

N.P. A Pap test is a test in your uterus when we look for (unintelligible) at the opening of your uterus. Do you think you've ever had one of those?

P. I might have had one years ago, but that was before they took my, ah . . .

N.P. You had a hysterectomy?

P. Yeah.

N.P. Okay, so you should have a pelvic exam even if you had a hysterectomy. You can't get cancer of the uterus because you don't have a uterus, but we should take a look in your vagina and see if, it would be very unusual for you to have a problem, but we should do a Pap, do that next time, another visit.

P. Okay.

N.P. And check your breasts. In fact, we could do that today. I'm not real busy. Would you like to do that today, or would you like to do it another time?

P. I think I'll come back.

N.P. Do you check your breasts at home?

P. Sometimes. If I think about it. Not very often.

N.P. Okay. It's a good thing to do once a month.

P. (Laughs.)

N.P. Do you have a calendar that you check daily?

P. No.

N.P. Maybe you need to put a sign over your bed to remind you. The first of the month//

P. //I do it but not too often.

N.P. Okay. Well it still needs to be done, and we should do a pelvic exam. Okay. Do you have sex with anyone now?

The topics of prevention and how to care for oneself, while central to the mission of primary care, are all too often left uncovered in medical consultations. Nurse practitioners claim that their commitment to these topics is, in large part, the distinguishing feature in the way they deliver care. In addition, as we have seen, these topics provide a rich site for the negotiation of social/ideological assumptions, which carry significant medical consequences. Here, assumptions about women and sexuality influence the way a potential medical problem is dealt with differently from the way such problems were dealt with in the medical consultations.

All too often women of Pat's age are assumed to be either sexually exclusive or sexually inactive—ideological assumptions that were clearly evident in Doctor Johnson's consultation with Muriel. Because cervical cancer is positively associated with sexual activity—specifically early intercourse or multiple partners—if older women are without symptoms and are assumed to be celibate or monogamous, they are not treated as if they are at risk. If they are not at risk, they do not need to be screened.

They do not need to have routine Pap smears. This assumption is clearly at odds with the statistics gathered by the U.S. National Center for Health Statistics (compare Fisher 1986).

Claudia does not make these assumptions. In the absence of symptoms and with an older patient who is living alone and has described herself as socially isolated, she checks the file for laboratory evidence of a recent Pap smear. When she finds none, she asks whether Pat has had a Pap test since becoming a patient of this clinic. After she explains what a Pap smear is, she learns that Pat may have had one prior to her hysterectomy. Although Claudia does not explore why a hysterectomy was performed,[3] she does take this opportunity to educate Pat about reproductively related topics —the need for Pap smears even after a hysterectomy.

After explaining that Pat should have regular Pap smears and do routine self-examinations of her breast, Claudia offers her two options. She explains that since she has the time, she could do a breast exam and a Pap smear on this visit, or Pat could return for these procedures. Pat chooses to return, to have them at another time. Claudia also stresses the importance of regular breast self-examinations—a topic Pat has difficulty with. When asked whether she examines her breasts regularly, Pat says, "Sometimes. If I think about it. Not very often." And after Claudia offers several suggestions for how she might remember to think about and do them more often, Pat concludes, "I do it but not too often." Claudia takes the hint, sums up, and changes the topic.

There are some interesting contrasts here. In the previous case the patient's presenting complaint—vaginal bleeding seven years after a hysterectomy—sent a strong signal about cancer. Even though the doctor assumed that as an older, recently widowed woman Muriel was not sexually active, he performed a Pap smear—a diagnostic test for cancer. He did so without taking a sexual history, explaining what he was going to do, or getting the patient's permission to proceed. After the fact he told Muriel that a Pap smear is necessary even after a hysterectomy.

In this case, although there are no explicit symptoms of cancer and the patient is also older (fifty-four years old), unmarried, and socially isolated, the nurse practitioner does not just assume that she is celibate. She asks, "Do you have sex with anyone now?" In my experience this is an amazing question. It does not recirculate hegemonic assumptions about black women and sexuality (they are rampantly sexual), about middle-aged women and sexuality (they are sexually inactive), or about heterosexuality (only men and women engage in sexual relations together). The "anyone" is self-consciously gender neutral. Moreover, by locating the question in a particular moment in time, "now," the nurse practitioner does not depict sexual activity as something one engages in until a certain age or a specific point in the life cycle. Instead, a woman's sexuality is refigured as much more flexible. Sometimes one is sexually active and at other times not.

Even though Pat does not answer the question about her current sexual activity, Claudia goes on to discuss the importance of routine Pap smears as a preventive health measure. She asks whether the patient would rather have a Pap smear now or later. Here the nurse practitioner neither lets dominant cultural assumptions color her clinical practice nor imposes her will on the patient without providing an explanation or seeking her permission.

Although it is impossible to know for sure, it seems reasonable to suggest that, in the absence of symptoms, preventive procedures like Pap smears and breast exams are less likely to be performed when patients are desexualized because of age or marital status. The manner in which preventive procedures are dealt with in the cases here provides some support for this supposition. In the end both Muriel and Pat have Pap smears, but Muriel's is diagnostically indicated by her presenting complaint and Pat's is not. More important, even though breast cancer is quickly becoming the number one killer of women, with Muriel breast exams were neither discussed nor performed. By contrast both preventive procedures are discussed with Pat. She is encouraged to do routine self-examinations and to return to the clinic for a Pap smear and breast exam.

Doctor and nurse practitioner have each asked their patients to return to take care of matters they leave unfinished in this examination. However, both the matters left unaddressed and the consequences are quite different. In the medical encounter, during an initial visit for an urgent medical problem, Muriel repeatedly tried to talk about the social/biographical context of her life. But she was unsuccessful. The doctor insistently channeled the discussion toward medical topics. However, in the closing moments of the consultation, he suggested that Muriel make another appointment to discuss the emotional issues she had been raising. She never did in the years that I followed her file.

In the nursing consultation, during a routine visit for chronic medical problems and in the absence of symptoms, the nurse practitioner initiates a discussion about the need for routine Pap smears and regular breast examinations. After this discussion, she offers Pat a choice about when to do these preventive procedures. Pat chooses not to do them now. In the years I followed her case, Pat made the same choice on several subsequent visits. But because Claudia had an ongoing relationship with her and could continue to raise the topic and educate her, eventually Pat made an appointment and had a Pap smear and a breast examination.

Even though both women are poor, the differences in their behavior cannot be explained in economic terms alone, especially because clinic funds are available to help defray the cost of subsequent visits. More likely, both what is deferred and the context in which it is deferred contribute to the patient's behavior. For Muriel this was a first visit to a new clinic and a new doctor. Pat has an ongoing relationship both at the clinic and with her provider. Moreover, the issues Doctor Johnson and Claudia Sussen defer are not of the same order, and they have been dealt with differently. Given Muriel's presenting complaint, a Pap smear is not optional, but discussing the troubles in her life seems to be. Doctor Johnson does the diagnostic work-up suggested by her presenting complaint, but after consistently avoiding her more social/biographical concerns, he asks her to come back to discuss them on another visit. Although Claudia also takes care of Pat's immediate medical problems, she discusses the need for preventive procedures and makes it possible for the patient to defer them to another visit. On subsequent visits the nurse practitioner continues to educate about the need for these procedures until she is finally successful.

It seems entirely possible that both the nature of the topics deferred—social/biographical talk and preventive medical procedures—and the ways the topics have been handled initially—consistently avoided and repeatedly discussed—contribute to the patient's subsequent behavior. It was quite reasonable for Muriel to decide not to make another appointment to discuss the social/biographical topics avoided on this visit. Since she brought these topics into the conversation on several occasions without success, she had no experience on which to base a decision to return, no experience that suggested that the doctor could or would discuss the troubles in her life at another time. Pat, by contrast, has all the experience she needs to know that Claudia will continue encouraging her to have a Pap smear and breast exam.

But factors other than the way Doctor Johnson consistently prioritized medical topics—a priority reflected in his take-care-of-medical-business-first attitude—also contributed to the patient's decision. The doctor consistently recirculated a social/ideological conception of Muriel as a less-than-competent patient—an assumption that might have become a self-fulfilling prophecy. If he persistently located her as less than competent and the social/biographical topics she introduced as irrelevant, there was no reason to discuss the context of her life. Because he did not take her concerns seriously, she had no incentive to return to talk about what she had not been able to discuss on the first visit.

The nursing encounter provides a different decision-making context. Claudia has taken care of medical business, but she has not bifurcated the medical and the social/biographical into separate and unrelated realms. Moreover, she does not consistently present Pat as incompetent. Most of the time she treats her as quite competent. Even if she presents Pat as a competent patient on only some occasions, this attitude may become a motivating factor, making a different decision likely. Claudia can provide the information Pat needs to make her decision, give her the space to do so, and trust that in time she will.

But however the differences in these cases are understood, it seems perfectly clear that in both the medical and the nursing consultation social/ideological assumptions penetrate the discussion of complaints that have been easily coded as medical. This conclusion emerges even more clearly in the next set of exchanges.

> N.P. Okay. Well it still needs to be done, and we should do a pelvic exam. Okay. Do you have sex with anybody now?
> P. No.
> N.P. Is that all right with you?
> P. Yes, it's fine.
> N.P. Do you ever masturbate? Do you know what that means?
> P. Masturbate (very softly).
> N.P. Do you ever touch your vagina or clitoris?
> P. In the bath. In the water.
> N.P. Just in the bath, in the water? You never touch yourself for sexual enjoyment? Some people do that.
> P. I wouldn't know what to do. (Laughs.)
> N.P. You wouldn't know what to do?
> P. (Laughs.) Uh uh! (Shakes her head no.)
> N.P. We used to be told that that was a bad thing to do, that we shouldn't excite ourselves sexually. (P. Oh yeah?) People now know that that's an okay thing to do.
> P. Oh yeah?
> N.P. Yeah. Some people who don't have partners, who aren't having sex with a partner, will excite themselves sexually, and that's an okay thing to do.
> P. Oh, yeah! Maybe I need to do that. I ain't had none in over two years. (Laughs.)
> N.P. (Laughs.) Well, listen, you could!

P. Maybe I need to do that! (Laughs//)

N.P. // You had a partner two years ago?

P. (Still laughing.) Lord have mercy.

N.P. What?

P. (Still laughing.) Ain't that crazy. Love is as queer as the day is long.

N.P. I don't think that's crazy.

P. Ah, dear, dear, yeah, it's been a long time since I had sex with anyone. You know? (N.P. Uh huh.) I even got so I don't even think about it.

N.P. Do you ever think you might get another relationship again?

P. I think, well, I don't know. What I, to tell. I'm going to tell you the truth. All these men around here, all they're looking for is sex and money. And, see, I don't have that, and I don't play around. (N.P. Um hum.) And I just would rather leave them alone.

N.P. So you haven't found anybody that you're particularly interested in spending time with? (P. No-o-o.) Well, that's okay.

P. No, I've never met somebody like that. They just mess up your life in the meeting. I don't care for that; I'm too old for that.

N.P. Is that, is that what happened with your husband? You were too old to have your life messed up, but I don't think you're too old to have a relationship.

P. I'm too old to have my life messed up, that's for sure (N.P. Um hm.), and again I see too much happening.

N.P. If someone you liked came along, would you be open to trying to be in a relationship?

P. I'm, I might. But it would probably take me a while. He'll have to prove to me that he, he cared; otherwise nothing doing.

N.P. You've been hurt before.

P. Yeah, that's right.

N.P. It sounds like you're reaching out to your friends right now, and that's great.

P. Yeah.

N.P. I'm glad to hear that.

These are the last major exchanges of the consultation. After the topic shift that ends this section, Claudia prescribes a new medication to treat the troublesome scab dealt with earlier and closes the consultation by telling Pat that she would like her "to come back in a week and let me take a look."

As the discussion in this last section unfolds, the social/ideological tensions discussed earlier are illuminated quite clearly. These tensions are between a discourse that reinscribes an asymmetrical medical relationship and one that offers a more symmetrical alternative to it, and between those discourses that recirculate dominant cultural assumptions about women and sexuality and those that provide a more oppositional understanding.

Claudia has not assumed that because Pat is a fifty-four-year-old divorced woman who has described herself as socially isolated, that she is either celibate or monogamous. She thus resists dominant cultural assumptions—social/ideological assumptions—about the appropriate sexual appetites of older unmarried women. From this perspective she again raises questions about the social/biographical context of Pat's life. She asks whether Pat is having sex with anyone now. When Pat responds "no," she asks, "Is that all right with you?" Pat responds, "Yes, it's fine."

Unlike Doctor Johnson, Claudia seems to have no trouble talking about sexuality, and this has an influence on her clinical practice. She does not assume that Pat is familiar with, or accepts, the sexual practices available to her. From her position as a primary-care provider and the dominant interactional partner, the nurse practitioner moves to educate the patient. She indicates that there is another choice besides sexual intercourse or celibacy—a choice that is certainly at odds with dominant cultural assumptions. She asks, "Do you ever masturbate? Do you know what that means?"

Pat does not answer this question. Instead, she softly repeats the word *masturbate*. In the absence of a response, Claudia explains that masturbation means touching your vagina or clitoris. Pat still does not seem clear about what Claudia is trying to convey. She responds by acknowledging that she touches herself when she bathes. But touching oneself for cleanliness is not the same as touching for sexual pleasure, a point that Claudia makes quite clear when she asks, "Just in the bath, in the water? You never touch yourself for sexual enjoyment? Some people do that." Pat laughs and says that she would not know what to do.

Although it does not seem hard for Claudia to discuss sexuality and even masturbation, this is not the case for Pat. The way she softly repeats the forbidden word, masturbate, and laughs gives voice to her discomfort. Even though Pat has not described her feelings, Claudia picks up on them, and, speaking in an oppositional voice, she tells Pat that although people used to say it was a bad thing to sexually excite "ourselves," people now know "that's an okay thing to do."

Pat begins to lose her reticence. She indicates that she is paying close attention to what Claudia is telling her by saying, "Oh, yeah?" In so doing she provides an opportunity for Claudia to reassure her again—an opportunity Claudia takes. "Yeah. Some people who don't have partners, who aren't having sex with a partner, will excite themselves sexually, and that's an okay thing to do." Throwing caution to the wind, Pat again says, "Oh yeah!" and continues, "Maybe I need to do that. I ain't had none in over two years." Pat's acknowledgement that perhaps she could masturbate since she "ain't had none in over two years" seems to embarrass her. Pat laughs. Claudia laughs with her and at the same time encourages her. She says, "Well, listen, you could!"

While still laughing, Pat continues exploring the possibility that she could masturbate—an exploration that is interspersed with comments from Claudia. But it is Pat's talk that is most interesting. Pat goes on to say, "Maybe I need to do that!" "Lord have mercy." "Ain't that crazy. Love is as queer as the day is long." You can hear how Pat is processing an alternative definition of her sexuality—a definition that might make pleasuring herself a legitimate option, and you can hear Claudia supporting her. As their laughter dies away, Claudia says, "I don't think that's crazy." Pat seems to accept her reassurance saying, "Ah, dear, dear, yeah, it's been a long time since I had sex with anyone. You know? I even got so I don't even think about it."

Both of the social/ideological tensions I mentioned earlier are apparent here. On the one hand, Claudia foregrounds her status as a medical provider. She initiates the discussions about both sexual intercourse and masturbation and defines the situation. From her location as medical expert, she declares that it is okay to masturbate and encourages Pat to do so. In doing so, she enacts the characteristic asymmetry of the provider-patient relationship and recirculates dominant assumptions about the status of the provider and patient. As she does so, she speaks an oppositional discourse about older women and sexuality.

But, on the other hand, as the discussion continues, Claudia loses some of the distance her professional status affords. The way Claudia talks about masturbation positions her as a woman like Pat—a woman who understands the sexual mores of the dominant culture. This location undermines the characteristic asymmetry in the provider-patient relationship. When Claudia says, "*We* used to be told that it was a bad thing to do, that *we* shouldn't excite ourselves sexually," she repositions herself as a woman like Pat and distances herself from her professional status. Despite the differences between them, this language works to produce a solidarity based in women's common experiences.

This solidarity is very much in evidence as both women laugh. Claudia is not laughing at Pat. Claudia and Pat are laughing together. They are laughing at the discussion of a taboo topic—masturbation—and at the thought of a possible taboo action—pleasuring oneself sexually. Although in many significant ways Claudia and Pat are quite different, the solidarity they produce here also makes sense. Many of the differences are obvious. Claudia is the provider, and Pat is the patient. Claudia is white, and Pat is African American. Claudia is firmly middle class, and Pat is poor. Some are not quite so obvious. For example, at the time of this interview Claudia is married, and Pat is not.

However, differences notwithstanding, these women also share important cultural locations. Although Claudia is not an older woman, she is certainly more an age peer than not. She has been divorced and, for a period, socially isolated. But most important both Claudia and Pat are women who have come to maturity in a heterosexual and youth-oriented culture. And they share an understanding of that cultural space. Their joint laughter indicates that they both know that in the dominant culture it is not appropriate for women to engage in sexually explicit talk about how to pleasure themselves by masturbating. They also know that this topic is even more inappropriate for older women and during a professional encounter.

Here the social/ideological tension between dominant and alternative understandings about women and sexuality emerges most clearly. By bringing the topic of masturbation into the discussion, Claudia resists dominant cultural assumptions about women and sexuality. As Pat considers and then comes to accept the possibility that she can masturbate, she participates in the recirculation of this oppositional position. Their discussion offers an alternative in which women are depicted as having an active sexual interest even if they are middle-aged, unmarried, and socially isolated. And they have choices other than heterosexual intercourse or celibacy. Women are positioned as agents who can claim sexual pleasure for themselves and who will be supported in their choices by other women.

Although as a feminist I am all in favor of this kind of oppositional discourse, it would be a mistake to think that once Claudia and Pat have found each other in sisterhood, the differences between them disappear. The asymmetry usually associated with the provider-patient relationship does not just whither away. And dominant cultural assumptions about women and sexuality are not kept at bay for long. Instead, the discussion of the next topic—heterosexual relationships—once again displays a social/ideological tension between conflicting discourses.

After encouraging Pat to think about masturbation as an option, Claudia asks her whether she ever thinks about another relationship. Claudia suggests that masturbation need not permanently replace heterosexual intercourse. If masturbation is positioned as temporary, as a make-do method of sexual fulfillment, then a different message about women and sexuality is being sent. In it women masturbate only until another sexual partner can be found. While Claudia speaks about "partners" using a gender-neutral voice, Pat's response demonstrates that she hears male partners and heterosexual relationships. The way masturbation is refigured and heterosexual partner is reintroduced reclaim Claudia's status as the dominant interactional partner, while undermining the earlier oppositional discourse about women and sexuality. Pat resists, and a struggle ensues in a social/ideological register. Although the thought of pleasuring herself sexually appeals to Pat, the thought of a heterosexual relationship does not. She explains, "All these men around here, all they're looking for is sex and money. And, see, I don't have that, and I don't play around. And I just would rather leave them alone." Claudia tries again. She says, "So you haven't found anybody that you're particularly interested in spending time with? Well, that's okay."

Here, Claudia and Pat struggle over the asymmetrical nature of the provider-patient relationship as they argue about the likelihood of a satisfying heterosexual relationship. Pat claims that a relationship is not possible for her because all the available men are interested only in "sex and money." Given these interests, she would "rather leave them alone." Claudia tries to reposition Pat's response. It is not that all men are a bad risk but that Pat has not yet found the right man. She suggests that although it is all right to be choosy, Pat should keep looking until she finds a suitable man. I wonder whether this struggle is not also about race and class.[4] Is looking for a good man a somewhat different activity for a middle-class, white professional woman than it is for a poor, African American woman? Is Pat trying to convey this difference when she talks about men just wanting money and sex, when she claims she does not have money and she does not casually do sex?

As the encounter continues, so do the social/ideological struggles. Claudia presses for her definition of the situation, and Pat resists. Pat makes her position more explicit, saying that she has never met the right person. For her, "they just mess up your life in the meeting. I don't care for that; I'm too old for that." But Claudia does not accept her explanation. She counters by implying that although that may have been what happened with Pat's husband, it does not have to be the case in all relationships. Pat may be too old to have her life disrupted, but a good relationship is possible at any age. For Pat, however, a relationship seems to go hand in hand with having her life upset. She restates her position: "I'm too old to have my life messed up, that's for sure, and again I see too much happening."

Claudia, talking about the social/biographical context of Pat's life, raises the topic of relationships and pushes Pat to look for a good man. Even though relationships have "messed up" Pat's life in the past, Claudia argues that they need not do so in the future. In Claudia's definition of the situation one is never too old to find Mister Right. Pat disagrees initially and continues to do so. But Claudia does not drop the topic. She modifies her position a little and tries again: "If someone you liked came along, would you be *open* to trying to be in a relationship?" Pat agrees that she might. "But it would probably take me a while." Finally, Claudia and Pat reach a tentative and conditional agreement "He'll have to prove to me that he, he cared; otherwise nothing doing"—and this topic is dropped. Claudia has pressed to have her definition of the situation prevail. She insists that for Pat a heterosexual relationship is possible and, by implication, desirable. Pat resists but is not successful. Both women are unrelenting until Claudia moves to break the deadlock by asking for a tentative and conditional agreement.

But the agreement is not nearly as interesting as the social/ideological struggle has been. Although Claudia and Pat struggle in a social/ideological register, their discussion is taking place in a medical setting and on Claudia's terms. She initiates the topic of relationship, reframes it, pushes her definition of the situation, and obtains a tentative and conditional agreement. In so doing she enacts the asymmetry characteristic of the provider-patient relationship. The woman-to-woman symmetry of the earlier discussion of masturbation is replaced—perhaps with class and race overtones. Claudia relocates herself as the dominant interactional partner and repositions Pat as the subordinate patient. From this position of institutional authority, Claudia abandons her earlier oppositional discourse and circulates hegemonic notions about women and sexuality. Although on some occasions a woman can pleasure herself sexually, her proper place is in a heterosexual relationship.

These are interesting struggles. They reinforce the view that social/ideological struggles over competing discourses do not take place just between provider and patient—a view that was also apparent in the medical consultation discussed in the previous chapter. Doctor Johnson took a consistent discursive position, but

Muriel did not. She struggled over competing definitions of women and sexuality. Pat takes a consistent position—heterosexual relationships are trouble—but Claudia does not. When she speaks about masturbation, she circulates an oppositional discourse and speaks from an alternative location—as a woman like Pat. But when Claudia talks about heterosexual relationships, she speaks a hegemonic discourse and talks from a position of institutional authority.[5] I wonder whether Claudia's oppositional discourse—her movement away from the asymmetry of the provider-patient relationship and from dominant understandings about women and sexuality—calls this more hegemonic enactment into play.

But although there is no definitive way to know what produces Claudia's struggle, we do know that both the social/ideological struggle with herself and the struggles with Pat take place during discussions of the social/biographical context of Pat's life. We also know that Pat does not just passively accept either Claudia's authority or her definition of the situation. She resists, and although she does not prevail, her resistance shapes subsequent interactions. Claudia reframes the way she is talking about relationships to generate a conditional agreement.

Taken together, the four cases discussed demonstrate that whether complaints are marked as social psychological or coded as medical, social talk is certainly done. Yet this social talk is much more complex than it at first appears. The doctors consistently avoid the social/biographical context of patients' lives, but the nurse practitioners do not. However, encouraging patients to talk about their lives neither erases the characteristic asymmetry of the provider-patient relationship nor automatically humanizes it.

Moreover, in each encounter, whether discussions are held in social or medical voices, social/ideological assumptions invade them and undermine the presumed neutrality of the provider-patient relationship. In each case conflicting social/ideological discourses about the identities of providers and patients and the nature of the medical relationship are struggled over. In these struggles patients often resist. Although sometimes this resistance is successful, in the end providers' definitions prevail.

Despite the similarities in all four consultations, there are also important differences. These differences suggest that medical and nursing encounters provide different sites for the delivery of health care, the negotiation of identity, and the production of knowledge. In these sites women's medical and more social wounds seem to be cared for differently. In the next chapter I explore this contention more systematically.

SEVEN

INSTITUTIONAL PATTERNS OF INTERPRETATION

I chose the two sets of cases just discussed to compare how the social and the medical function in provider-patient encounters. Nurse practitioners claim to provide a system of care that combines the psychological and the physiological—caring and curing. Yet we have little qualitative empirical data about what nurse practitioners actually do in examining rooms or how it compares with what doctors do in similar situations. In addition, although many researchers have documented a medical relationship characterized by an asymmetry between provider and patient and by the nearly total exclusion of the social/biographical context of patients' lives (Mishler 1984, Fisher 1986, Todd 1989), we neither know whether nurses practice in the same way nor agree theoretically about how to remedy these problems. The discussion in the previous four chapters, then, was intended to shed light on caring as clinical practice and as a theoretical remedy to the troubles that all too frequently plague the provider-patient relationship—to shed light on whether nurses do it differently and, if they do, how to account for those differences.[1]

The previous four chapters were organized to compare the ways nurse practitioners and doctors provide care to women patients whose complaints are easily marked as social psychological or coded as medical. My goals were both to display how doctors and nurse practitioners provide care and to address whether the presenting complaint shapes the way they do so. The central questions here were whether diffuse complaints, where no organic pathology is found, provide a more fertile site for the discussion of the social/ biographical context of patients lives and, if they do, whether they do so in the same way for both doctors and nurses. Or, by contrast, do complaints that are accepted as an indication of organic pathology provide an equally fruitful site for these discussions? And, in addition, I wanted to explore whether doctors or nurse practitioners or both of them just identify the pathology and treat it in a value-free and objective manner or whether social/ideological assumptions penetrate the presumed neutrality of provider-patient discussions, and if so, how.

In the four cases I found important similarities. Whether complaints were coded as medical or marked as social psychological, whether the social/biographical contexts of patients' lives were discussed or not, social/ideological assumptions penetrated the discussions as often for nurse practitioners as for doctors. Furthermore, there was no evidence that encouraging patients to speak in a social voice about their lives eliminated the characteristic asymmetry of the provider-patient relationship. Yet the way this asymmetry was enacted—whether or not providers made space for patients to talk about their lives—and the nature of the social/ideological talk were quite different in the nursing and medical encounters.

These differences are far from insignificant. They influence the way health care is delivered and contribute to the production of knowledge and the negotiation of identities. They also have important implications for both nursing's claim that a system of care remedies the troubles in provider-patient encounters and for the either/or theoretical accounts about the nature of the provider-patient relationship and how to fix it—accounts like those by Mishler (1984), Silverman (1987), and Waitzkin (1983), which were discussed in Chapter One.

In this chapter I change the focus of my analytic gaze. Instead of comparing how care is delivered by doctors and nurse practitioners when patients' presenting complaints are different, I treat the medical and nursing consultations as sites for the production of knowledge and the negotiation of identity and compare how in these sites institutional patterns of interpretation are produced. Here, I am indebted to Nancy Fraser (1989). Although she is talking about the institution of social work and I am discussing the institutions of medicine and nursing, in each case there are similar kinds of struggles over conflicting interpretations of women's needs and over whose interpretation is authoritative. These struggles take place in a social/ideological register, and the potential stakes are high. At stake are understandings about professional and gendered identities, notions about class and race, as well as ideas about women, work, and the nuclear family and women, age, and sexuality—in other words, the way dominant cultural assumptions are reproduced or undermined. This shift in analytic focus lays the foundation for subsequent discussions in Chapter Eight, where I reframe the discussion about the nature of the provider-patient relationship and reformulate either/or theoretical debates.

SETTING THE STAGE

To explore how medicine and nursing are sites for the production of knowledge and the negotiation of identity, I return to the initial moments of the encounter. In these moments the stage is set.

There are striking differences and equally striking similarities in the doctor-patient and the nurse practitioner–patient relationship, and these differences and similarities are reiterated, albeit in slightly different form, with both complaints marked as social psychological and those coded as medical. Doctors and nurse practitioners each walk into examining rooms carrying the patient's medical file and wearing clear markers of their professional status—white coats and stethoscopes. By doing so, all the providers position themselves as medical experts and enact the institutional authority so often associated with this location.

After establishing their professional status, doctors and nurses rely on or distance themselves from this status differently. Doctors Aster and Johnson enter examining rooms where the patients, Wendy and Muriel, are sitting on the examining tables waiting for them. The encounters begin as the doctors stand looking down at the patients. In each case, doctors begin the consultation in ways that foreground the asymmetry of the provider-patient relationship, recirculating their professional status and their identities as doctors. And, in so doing, they position patients as subordinate others.

The nurse practitioners, Katherine Heinz and Claudia Sussen, also enter examining rooms wearing the marks of their professional status, which reiterates their identities as medical experts. However, whereas in the medical consultation doctors consistently fore-ground one version of reality—a version in which they are domi-nant and patients are subordinate—nurse practitioners do not. They simultaneously undermine their professional status, minimiz-ing the difference between professional and layperson, between provider and patient. These institutional patterns of interpretation recur repeatedly. Where in the medical consultations both patients wait for their doctors while seated on the examining tables, in the nursing encounters both patients wait for their nurse practitioners while seated on chairs. Where both doctors stand and look down at the patients, both nurse practitioners sit across from patients and look directly at them.

Space is consciously arranged by the nurse practitioners. When they set up their examining rooms, they make sure that there are two chairs in the room so that patients have something other than the examining table to sit on. Although the doctors have the same opportunities, they make no similar arrangements. They seem to take no interest in spatial arrangement; however, they position themselves in significant ways that reproduce their professional identities and the asymmetry characteristic of medical consulta-tions. But the nurses do not.

When the complaint is coded as medical, there is an additional difference between the doctor and the nurse practitioner. Before Doctor Johnson sees Muriel, she is prepared to meet him by a nurse. These preparations entail getting out of her street clothes and into a paper gown that opens down the back. Although it might be argued that the medical nature of the complaint produces this behavior, there is no similar behavior in the nursing encounter where the complaint is coded as medical. Sitting dressed and look-ing eye-to-eye with your provider sends quite a different message from sitting on an examining table in a hospital gown while your provider stands in front of you in street clothes and looks down at you.

Overall, these differences have less to do with presenting com-plaints and more to do with the production of meaning and the negotiation of identity. Even in the opening moments of the encounter, doctors repetitively reiterate their professional status—reinscribing the category of professional expert and an asymmetrical medical relationship. Although nurse practitioners enact their professional status as well as the nature of the professional relationship in a similar way, they also undermine both. Nursing interactions do not simply reproduce a logic in which providers are dominant and patients are not. However, they do not abandon this logic either. After all, nurse practitioners do set the interactional stage by reiterating their professional identities and an asymmetrical provider-patient relationship or by distancing themselves from them.

In nursing encounters, then, from the opening moments forward there is tension between discourses that reinscribe and those that undermine nurses' professional identities and the characteristic asymmetry of the provider-patient relationship—a tension not present in medical consultations. This tension both leaves the way open for providers and patients to renegotiate their identities as well as the nature of the professional relationship and generates a struggle in a social/ideological register—a struggle that is evident regardless of the presenting complaint.[2] Establishing solidarity based on common understandings about gender, class, sexuality, and age dismantles professional status and undermines the hierarchy associated with a professional encounter.[3]

ESTABLISHING SOLIDARITY

During the opening moments and throughout the consultation doctors make no attempt to establish solidarity or to minimize status differences. Doctors Aster and Johnson and patients Wendy and Muriel remain doctor and patient, man and woman throughout the consultations, particularly so in the encounter between Doctor Johnson and Muriel. Although they are both Appalachians, their shared location in this region does not produce solidarity.

In the nursing encounters the situation is quite different. Providers and patients establish and maintain a kind of solidarity. Katherine calls on her status as a woman to legitimate Prudence's anger and frustration and to support her reluctance to be contained by traditional domestic arrangements. She assures Prudence that she and all the women she knows would not do well in the situation Prudence describes. In addition, after encouraging Prudence to talk with friends about the troubles in her life, Katherine acknowledges a shared hesitancy to wash and air dirty linens in public—a class-based hesitancy.

The discussion of sexuality provides similar opportunities for Claudia. Although nurse practitioner and patient are different in many ways, both are women and neither is young. Using these shared locations, Claudia produces a kind of solidarity based on their common understandings as older women who have come to maturity in a heterosexual, youth-oriented culture.[4] In this culture it is commonly understood that sex is for the young and that self-stimulation is not the preferred mode. Sex is understood as heterosexual intercourse—an understanding widely circulated in dominant discourses. By engaging in sexually explicit talk, encouraging Pat to pleasure herself sexually by masturbating, and generating Pat's enthusiasm for such actions, Claudia violates shared normative understandings and circulates alternatives. As she educates Pat and garners her agreement, Claudia also establishes a kind of solidarity between them.

Establishing solidarity, or failing to do so, shapes the medical and the nursing encounters. In these cases doctors continuously reiterate their professional identity and in this process reinscribe the identities of doctor and patient, man and woman. By speaking only as doctors, they do not establish solidarity. Instead, they consistently recirculate a hierarchical relationship.

Although nurse practitioners speak as health-care providers and locate their interactions in an asymmetrical professional relationship, they also position themselves in a community of women—albeit different communities of women—and thereby produce a kind of solidarity not in evidence in medical encounters. Gender is at the heart of these productions; however, class and age as well as notions about sexuality and heterosexuality also play their parts. On the basis of these shared locations, nurse practitioners distance themselves from the institutional authority and interactional dominance associated with their professional status and offer an alternative. However, doing so sets the stage for future struggles.[5]

PRODUCING COMPETENT OR
INCOMPETENT PATIENTS

Different institutional patterns of interpretation are evident in other ways as well. From the opening moments of the medical encounter and throughout, Doctors Aster and Johnson send a consistent message about Wendy's and Muriel's competence as patients: they are not competent. This message is produced both in what is said and in the way it is said. Both doctors ask their patients to repeat information they have presented and check and recheck their presentations. In addition, Doctor Aster implies that Wendy does not competently manage her emotions. She is not sick; her out-of-control emotions have caused her symptoms and brought her to the doctor's office. And Doctor Johnson implies that Muriel has not used birth control competently.

In each consultation there is an exception. Doctor Aster situates Wendy as competent because she followed her husband's directions. When Wendy felt as though she were going to pass out, her husband told her to put her head between her knees and breathe more slowly, and she did. She may be an overly emotional woman who is not competent in her own right, but she can competently follow the directions of others—in this example, her more competent husband. Similarly, Doctor Johnson establishes Muriel as competent for identifying a potentially serious medical symptom and seeking medical attention to diagnosis and treat it. Here, the exception may be related to the nature of the presenting complaint—a complaint coded as medical and potentially quite serious. However, although Muriel competently got herself to the doctor, once in the examining room her everyday competence was insufficient to the medical task at hand.

These exceptions may appear minor, but they contribute to the clear social/ideological messages being sent. Both women are portrayed as incompetent in their own lives and unable to report their medical histories competently, to talk credibly about their lives. These messages reinscribe hegemonic understandings about women and patients. In addition, by consistently locating the patients as less than competent, the doctors just as consistently promote others—husbands and doctors—as the competent ones. In so doing, they recirculate their gendered and professional identities as they promote the authority of male others, and they reproduce the hierarchical arrangements of the nuclear family and the provider-patient relationship as well as the "proper" place for women in both.

In these consultations the doctors depict themselves as competent not only to diagnose and treat but to define how patients should live their lives. If Wendy does not work in the paid labor force and instead stays home and takes care of her family, she will not somatize. And Muriel can cure her medical symptoms and be a better woman if her sexual activity is consistent with her age and her current stage of life—her recent widowhood. These definitions of the situation reproduce hegemonic understandings of appropriate gendered behavior. In them women are defined by their age and their heterosexual domestic arrangements.

The nursing encounters are different. With few exceptions, Katherine and Claudia speak a social/ideological discourse that sends the message that Prudence and Pat are competent both in their lives and in examining rooms. In sharp contrast with the medical consultations, where patients' definitions of the situation are contested, both patients in the nursing encounters define their medical problems. Prudence diagnoses herself, and Pat tells Claudia how to remove the scab on her arm.

There is another important difference. In the medical encounters, emotions either are dismissed as not relevant to the discussion or are defined as out of control and located as the cause of the problem. In either case, if patients speak about their emotions from the social/biographical context of their lives, they run the very real risk of being reduced to these emotions, of being cast as overly emotional, out-of-control women and, on this basis, dismissed.

By contrast, in the nursing encounters both Prudence and Pat are encouraged to talk about the social/biographical context of their lives—to speak their emotions. Neither patient is presented as overly emotional or out of control. Nor are their emotions defined as the source of their problems. Instead, once spoken, their feelings about their lives are generally affirmed. This presentation is in opposition to, and undermines, dominant cultural understandings about gender.

Although in the nursing encounters patients are overwhelmingly positioned as competent, there is an exception. Early in the encounter Claudia asks Pat about the medications she has been taking. When an answer is not immediately forthcoming, she probes and Pat responds. Claudia evaluates this response, praising Pat for responding correctly. This evaluation looks like much of what occurs in the medical consultations; it produces a conception of the patient as a less-than-competent adult.[6]

In one other exchange in each of the nursing encounters questions about the patient's competence could arise. When Katherine presses for a divorce to solve the problems in Prudence's life and when Claudia pushes for a heterosexual relationship so that Pat does not have to rely solely on pleasuring herself through masturbation, both patients resist. Although they are not successful in changing the providers' definition of the situation to correspond with theirs, they do generate a struggle in a social/ideological register. The providers could invalidate the patients' responses by depicting them as overly emotional or less than competent, but they do not. After pushing for their definition of the situation and struggling, both providers suggest more moderate alternatives and reach compromise agreements with their patients.

There is a telling point to be made here. Although in both the nursing encounters patients are consistently represented as competent, in the encounter between Claudia and Pat there is an exception. Both this exception and the ways patients are able to resist, generate a struggle, and induce more moderate alternatives as the basis for a compromise agreement suggest that providers and patients do not speak in only one voice. Instead there is a conflict between discursive positions, which is reflected both on the single occasion Claudia locates Pat as incompetent and in the ways both providers respond to their patients' resistance by offering a compromise position.

The comparison between the exceptions that take place in the medical interactions and those that could have taken place in the nursing encounters but did not is also interesting. In the medical consultations the patients are represented as competent only when they seek or take the advice of husband or doctor. But in the nursing encounter, the patients are portrayed as competent in their own right. Perhaps reformulation and compromise are the logical result when patients are presented in this way.

Producing patients as competent or incompetent seems to have more to do with the status of the provider and the interactional site —a medical or a nursing encounter—than with the type of presenting complaint. However, in the medical consultation there is a strong relationship between these factors. Doctors Johnson and Aster persistently reproduce their professional identities and the asymmetrical nature of the medical relationship. From this perspective they bifurcate medical and social topics. They treat the medical and the social/biographical as discrete categories—either a complaint has a medical basis or it does not—and they prioritize the medical and dismiss the social/biographical.[7] In this context Doctor Johnson suggests that Muriel, with a complaint coded medical, has competently sought medical care. But Doctor Aster implies that Wendy, with a complaint coded social psychological, has been competent only in the way she has followed her husband's (medical) advice.

The consultations with nurse practitioners are more complex and more fluid than those with doctors. The nurse practitioners reproduce and undermine both their professional identities and the hierarchical nature of the provider-patient relationship. In this more open and multilayered context conflicting positions can coexist. From this perspective the medical and the social are not positioned as oppositional categories. The social/biographical context of patients lives is rendered as connected to, rather than separated from, the medical process of making a diagnosis and a treatment recommendation. In turn these medical tasks are seen to have consequences for patients' lived experiences. On this basis patients are treated as competent whether their complaints are located as social psychological or medical.

These differences are significant. Wendy and Muriel are almost exclusively located as less than competent, while Prudence and Pat are just as insistently positioned as competent patients and adult women in charge of their lives and their health care. The messages being sent have class and gender implications. However, the implication in the nursing consultation is almost always the antithesis of the message in the doctor-patient encounter. Although a message of competence would be unusual in most provider-patient consultations, it is even more striking in the consultation with Pat, who is a poor, African American woman.

Not only are institutional patterns of interpretation different in the medical and nursing encounters, but producing patients as competent or incompetent sets the stage for future struggles over whose interpretations are authoritative—struggles that, while different, also take place in a social/ideological register. In the medical relationship the way that patients are produced as competent and incompetent persistently reinscribes doctors' professional identities and the asymmetrical nature of the medical relationship. In the nursing relationship, by contrast, the way the nurse practitioners consistently represent Prudence and Pat as competent patients and women maximizes patients' voices as it both reinscribes and undermines the hierarchical nature of the health-care consultation and the characteristic asymmetry of provider-patient relationships.

THE STRUGGLE

Although they take different forms, there are social/ideological struggles in each of the encounters discussed. Providers and patients struggle over diagnosis and treatment—over the medical definition of the situation. Here, they are struggling with each other. There are also struggles over dominant and alternative definitions of women, work, the nuclear family, age, sexuality, and heterosexuality. Here, providers and patients struggle with themselves or with each other or both. In these social/ideological contests conflicting positions about the appropriate roles for women in today's society are the most visible. Because these conflicts are at the heart of what is different and what is the same in the medical and nursing encounters, I discuss them one at a time.

The Medical Consultation

Doctor Aster. In this encounter, while doctor and patient agree on the diagnosis, they disagree about the cause of the problem and how to treat it. The struggle begins as Wendy explains that she felt as though she were going to pass out and was nauseous that morning. Rather than exploring the medical symptom—nausea—Doctor Aster identifies Wendy's problem as social psychological.[8] In so doing he abandons the medical in favor of the social. He then narrowly and ideologically locates the social in the patient's domestic relations.

Without inquiring further about Wendy's nausea or doing a thorough physical examination, Doctor Aster places Wendy's problem in a conflict between her new motherhood role and her work in the paid labor force. This conflict generates stress, which causes her to hyperventilate. If she stops working and stays at home, her stress will be eliminated, and her medical condition will be cured. Wendy repeatedly struggles against this definition of the situation.

The struggle here is about whose interpretation is authoritative. For Doctor Aster the medical task is to identify whether a complaint is medical or social psychological in nature. Once he has identified it as social psychological, his differential diagnosis tries to find the cause for Wendy's symptoms and locates it in her domestic arrangements. Wendy does not separate the medical and the social in this way. For her the medical makes sense only in a social/biographical context, which the doctor systematically devalues. Although she struggles to insert information about her life into the discussion, she does not usually succeed.

Doctor Aster consistently marginalizes the social/biographical; however, he just as persistently inserts social/ideological messages into a presumably medical discussion. Once he locates the presenting complaint in Wendy's domestic arrangements, he bases his treatment recommendations on this diagnosis and thereby reinscribes dominant cultural assumptions about women, work, and the nuclear family. Wendy consistently resists the doctor's definition of the situation. For her the problem is more situational. Her husband has been away more than usual, increasing her work-force responsibilities at a time when she is unable to get a full night's sleep and is afraid that she is pregnant. It is not her out-of-control emotions that have caused her to hyperventilate but situationally specific life conditions. Because Wendy defines the situation differently than the doctor does, it is not surprising that she also resists his treatment recommendation—to stop working and stay at home.

Although Wendy resists both the way the doctor marginalizes the social/biographical context of her life and his social/ideological message about the cause of her presenting complaint and its treatment, she never prevails, and the medical costs are high. Doctor

Aster never adequately deals with the medical topics she raises. On more than one occasion she mentions nausea but to no avail. Finally she tells him that she thinks she is pregnant. Even though the doctor downplays the need for a pregnancy test, he provides one. However, he neither provides correct information about breastfeeding and contraception nor gives the patient any information about contraceptive options or a prescription for some form of birth control.

The social/ideological costs are equally significant. Wendy consistently speaks an oppositional discourse which circulates a competing definition of women, work, and the nuclear family. As she does so, she resists the way Doctor Aster locates the cause of her presenting complaint and his treatment recommendation. She also struggles to make her interpretations authoritative and thereby to undermine the characteristic asymmetry of the medical relationship —to reposition doctor and patient, man and woman in it. But she is unsuccessful. Although she and Doctor Aster have struggled, in the end dominant cultural assumptions about both domestic and medical relationships are reinscribed.

Doctor Johnson. In this encounter doctor and patient also struggle with each other. Although Muriel does not take exception to Doctor Johnson's diagnosis or his recommendation for treatment, she does resist the ways he defines several situations. She resists the way he portrays her as not competent to discuss her symptoms. She struggles against his depiction of her sexual activity as inappropriate for an older, recently widowed woman. And she opposes his question about keeping her house clean. Each struggle occurs in a social/ideological register, and in each the doctor circulates dominant cultural assumptions about women. Although Muriel resists repeatedly, before the encounter is over she justifies her actions and struggles with herself in ways that reinscribe the very discourses she has been resisting. But this struggle does not mean she has accepted the doctor's definition of the situation. Instead, it offers a particularly good view of the tensions between competing discursive positions.

In the opening moments of the encounter, as Muriel is discussing her presenting complaint, she explains that seven years earlier she had her uterus removed and now she is bleeding vaginally and she does not know why. Although she presents her complaint quite clearly, Doctor Johnson repeatedly checks to see whether she understands what she has said and whether she is reporting her medical history accurately. Thus, while discussing medical topics, he sends social/ideological messages with class and gender implications. Muriel resists but does not prevail.

Although the doctor has inserted social/ideological assumptions into a discussion of medical topics, as the consultation progresses doctor and patient struggle over Muriel's efforts to include social/ biographical information into the medical discussion. Doctor Johnson repeatedly asks narrowly focused medical questions. But for Muriel, as for Wendy, the medical is not so easily separated from a specific life context. Although she struggles to squeeze this information into the discussion, she is not successful. Each time Muriel tries to tell her story, Doctor Johnson moves the interview back toward narrowly defined medical topics.[9]

Although the discussion is about medical topics, doctor and patient struggle in a social/ideological register about the validity of Muriel's description of her symptoms. In these struggles the doctor prioritizes the medical, marginalizes the social/biographical, and transports social/ideological assumptions into the discussion. These dynamics are essentially unchanged when the topic is explicitly social—the patient's sexuality and her attention to housekeeping.

After prompting from me and with considerable discomfort, Doctor Johnson asks Muriel whether she has been sexually active since her husband's death. Although this question has clear medical ramifications, the doctor is asking for social/biographical information. But his question is not framed in ways that would encourage Muriel to talk about the social context of her life. It is, instead, framed as a narrow question for which a simple yes or no would suffice. Muriel resists this frame by saying that she is not as active as she was when her husband was alive. But she is not successful in broadening the discussion.

However, at the same time, both the way the doctor raises this topic and the way he talks about Muriel's current sexual activity send clear social/ideological messages. They suggest that Muriel's sexual activity is not appropriate for a recently widowed woman her age. Perhaps Muriel could explain her situation in ways that would ease his discomfort, perhaps not. But she is not given a chance to do so, and there are clear medical consequences. The doctor's discomfort influences his clinical practice. Doctor Johnson neither takes a sexual history nor tests for a range of sexually transmitted diseases. He never clarifies the distinction between a sexually transmitted infection and a venereal disease, leaving Muriel without the information she needs to explain to her man friend what she has and why he needs to be treated. And he allows Muriel to leave the office without determining how her friend will be treated—by Doctor Johnson or by someone else.

As always a lot is at stake in these struggles. Muriel has resisted both the way the doctor marginalizes the social context of her life and his social/ideological assumptions that her sexual behavior is inappropriate, but she has been unable to influence his definition of the situation. He continues to exclude the social context of her life and to circulate hegemonic assumptions about women.

Although Muriel seems comfortable with her sexual behavior and is able, on this topic, to resist the doctor's social/ideological definition of the situation, on other topics she is less secure. In these discussions she both displays her familiarity with dominant cultural assumptions about women and reinscribes them. Being portrayed as a sexually promiscuous bearer of a venereal disease is one such topic. Given the stigma associated with this, she refashions herself. She explains that she did not contract her sexually transmitted infection through sexual intercourse but through swimming. To preserve her identity as a good woman, she recirculates hegemonic understandings about women and sexuality.

On other topics—why she did not have more children and why she needed a hysterectomy—she justifies her behavior differently. She explains that her husband decided that they would have no more children when he saw how upset she was by her last pregnancy. And her doctor decided that she needed a hysterectomy because she had a "spot" that could be dangerous and he was afraid that she could not carry another pregnancy to term. Here she protects her identity as a good woman by having men make these critical decisions for her.[10] But the cost is high. She revivifies dominant cultural assumptions about men and women and about the nature of both medical and domestic relationships.

As the medical consultation is coming to a close, Doctor Johnson raises the topics that Muriel has been trying to discuss throughout it—the troubles in her life. Muriel tells him that there are lots of problems, and Doctor Johnson hears that she may be clinically depressed. He addresses this potential medical problem by inquiring about the way she keeps house. Muriel moves quickly to affirm that she is a good housekeeper. With this information Doctor Johnson concludes that she is not clinically depressed and loses interest. Ironically, the doctor's suggestion and Muriel's move to salvage her identity both foreclose the discussion she has been trying to stimulate and reinscribe dominant cultural assumptions about women and their domestic responsibilities.

Similarities and differences. In this consultation, just as in the encounter between Doctor Aster and Wendy, doctor and patient struggle over conflicting discourses, and these struggles have consistent themes. Although social/ideological assumptions penetrate the doctor's discussion, the patient's talk about the social/biographical is constrained. By locating the patient as a less-than-competent other, the doctor is repeatedly positioned as the dominant interactional partner, the person whose interpretation of the situation is authoritative. Although the patient repeatedly resists, she is not able to influence the doctor's definition of the situation, not even once. By marginalizing what the patient says about her life and invalidating her resistance, the doctor can circulate cultural assumptions in an unfettered manner, and these assumptions insistently revivify hegemonic understandings about women.

There are other similarities in the doctor-patient encounters. In both, a two-place logic seems to be operating in two slightly different ways. First, either the doctor is the dominant interactional partner, the medical expert, or he is not. And, if not, no other role seems to be available to him. Second, either a complaint is medical or it is not. And this definition structures the encounter. If the complaint is located as social psychological, the medical aspects of the consultation are largely abandoned. Wendy, for example, with a complaint marked as social psychological, has little success getting Doctor Aster to take her medical complaints seriously. By contrast, if the complaint is seen as medical, social topics are quite systematically neglected. Muriel, with a complaint coded as medical, has little success getting Doctor Johnson to treat her social concerns thoughtfully. And in both cases the doctor's clinical practice is undermined.

Although both consultations are characterized by struggles over conflicting discourses, the struggles are somewhat different. Doctor Aster and Wendy struggle over women, work, and the nuclear family. For Doctor Johnson and Muriel, the primary struggle is about women, age, and sexuality. Whereas for the whole encounter Doctor Aster speaks from one discursive position and Wendy almost as consistently speaks from another, conflicting one, this dichotomy is not as clear cut in the encounter between Doctor Johnson and Muriel. Doctor Johnson consistently speaks a hegemonic discourse that revivifies both his professional identity and dominant cultural assumptions about women. Muriel usually struggles against these messages, but at three different points in the consultation she speaks in ways that recirculate hegemonic understandings about women and domestic responsibilities, women and sexuality, and the gendered relationship between men and women. In so doing, she displays her own involvement with conflicting discursive positions.

The Nursing Consultation

Katherine Heinz. In this consultation nurse practitioner and patient do not struggle over many of the issues that are sites of contestation for doctors and their patients. Katherine and Prudence agree about the nature of the presenting complaint and its cause. With a complaint marked as social psychological, Katherine does not abandon medical topics, avoid a physical examination, or marginalize the context of Prudence's life. Instead, without making a sharp distinction between the medical and the social, she encourages the patient to talk about her life, and as Prudence does so, she diagnoses herself. Katherine agrees with her definition and legitimates it.

When provider and patient struggle, they do so over the best way to treat the problems that have been identified. In these struggles, although the topic is medical, the discussion is in a social register and does ideological work. While provider and patient talk about potential treatments, they also struggle over whose definition of the situation will prevail, whose interpretation is authoritative.

As Prudence describes the troubles in her life—troubles that have manifested themselves both in fatigue and in a lack of libido—she speaks a social/ideological discourse that circulates an alternate understanding about women, work, and the nuclear family. Katherine, locating herself as a woman like Prudence, supports her and in the process disrupts dominant assumptions about medical and domestic relationships.

Prudence feels trapped. She has gotten a job, and she has tried talking with her husband. After they struggle, things improve for a little while, only to return to normal all too quickly. Katherine seems to hear that Prudence has tried to make her marriage better, feels that she has failed, and is now so frustrated that she is somatizing. In response she makes her treatment recommendations—divorce and therapy—and makes them more than once. Prudence resists each time. She claims that her husband will not allow her to go for therapy and knows every move she makes. She also states that she is not ready to get divorced. She was married at fifteen and has always been a wife and mother. Here, Prudence and Katherine are struggling in a social/ideological register over conflicting discourses, with Katherine circulating an oppositional position and Prudence reinscribing hegemonic understandings about women's proper place in society.

Although Katherine does not challenge Prudence's definition of the situation, she brings all the authority of her medical expertise to bear and recommends divorce again. Prudence resists once more, but this time for economic reasons. Even though her resistance recirculates dominant assumptions about women's economic dependence on men, they reflect a structural reality. The feminization of poverty reveals all too clearly women's limited earning capacity. Katherine accepts her definition of the situation—accepts that neither divorce nor therapy is a treatment option. With these options blocked, Katherine modifies her position and suggests ways for Prudence to stay married but manage her stress better: talking with friends, running, and changing jobs so that she is no longer working next to her husband.

At first, Prudence resists these recommendations too. She claims that they will make her husband angry, and he will pout. Katherine points out that since her husband pouts anyway, she might as well do what is good for her, and talking with friends and running would be good for her. Prudence agrees with this compromise, and she thereby accepts Katherine's oppositional proposal that she stay married but take care of herself despite her husband's resistance.

Here, Katherine has located herself both as the medical expert with the institutional authority to interpret Prudence's needs and to recommend what is best for her and as a woman like Prudence. In so doing she produces and undermines her professional identity. But whether speaking as a provider or as a woman like Prudence, she consistently speaks an oppositional discourse that challenges dominant cultural assumptions about the most appropriate ways to be a woman, wife, and mother in today's society.

Prudence's position is not as consistent. She moves discursively from reproducing hegemonic understandings to resisting them and circulating alternatives. In so doing she struggles with herself and with Katherine. But, although they struggle, Katherine never challenges Prudence's description of her life. In the face of resistance Katherine modifies her treatment recommendation. Instead of sticking to her definition of the situation, she reformulates it and suggests an alternative. When Prudence resists again, Katherine helps her redirect that resistance toward her husband, and a compromise is reached.

Claudia Sussen. The encounter between Claudia and Pat looks more like the discussions between Katherine and Prudence than like the medical consultations. Even though the complaint is easily coded as medical, Pat does not have to struggle to include the social/biographical context of her life in the discussion. Whether talking about the iatrogenic potential of blood-pressure medicine or about social isolation, sexuality, masturbation, depression, or relationships, the nurse practitioner initiates and pursues social/biographical information. She and Pat move easily between the medical and the social/biographical and have a similar flexibility in the ways they relate to each other—as provider and patient and as women who share certain social locations. Nevertheless, they struggle.

Although Claudia and Pat do not struggle about what caused the presenting complaint or how to diagnose it, like Katherine and Prudence they struggle over the most appropriate treatment. These struggles are over whose interpretation of the situation will prevail. And each does social/ideological work. The struggle over whether to remove the scab with Vaseline or water is also about the patient's and the provider's status. Both the decision-making process and the outcome are quite unusual, especially with a lower-class African American patient. Pat presents herself as medically competent, challenging Claudia's definition of the situation and the characteristic asymmetry of the provider-patient relationship. And she does so successfully. Claudia provides care in accordance with Pat's demands and defends her medical decision as well as her competence as a provider. Not only is the provider-patient relationship refigured, but an alternative discourse about the patient is circulated as well—a discourse with clear gender, racial, and class implications.

After a discussion of masturbation and perhaps because of it, Claudia initiates the topic of heterosexual relationships, and a struggle ensues. Just as Claudia has encouraged Pat to masturbate, she now encourages her to seek a relationship with a man. But whereas Pat found masturbation appealing, she has no similar response to this suggestion. She informs Claudia that all the men she knows, or knows about, just want sex and money. And she has no money and is unwilling to participate in casual sexual relations. Furthermore, in her opinion, and based on what she sees in her community, men just mess up women's lives, and she does not want her life messed up in this way.

These are perfectly clear statements; however, Claudia does not accept Pat's definition of the situation, does not accept her interpretation of her life and her needs as authoritative. Instead, she brings all the authority of her professional status and any good will she has established to bear and pushes to have Pat agree that she needs a man in her life and will look for one. Here, Claudia recirculates her professional identity as she reinscribes hegemonic understandings about women and heterosexual relationships.

Although they have struggled hard, neither woman can convince the other. After repeated unsuccessful attempts, Claudia reformulates her request and asks Pat whether, if a good man came along, she would be open to a potential relationship. And Pat agrees to this tentative and conditional compromise position.

Similarities and differences. Claudia and Katherine each positions herself as the person whose interpretation is authoritative, recirculating her professional identity. She knows her patient's needs better than the patient does herself. Although neither practitioner's recommendations are, strictly speaking, treatments, they are prescriptions for how Prudence and Pat should live their lives. But at the same time that these providers reproduce the asymmetry characteristic of the provider-patient relationship, they also dismantle it.

After a struggle Katherine and Claudia both accept their patients as experts on their own lives. And, in addition, Claudia accepts Pat as the expert on a medical topic—her scab. She thereby locates Pat as a woman like herself, undermining her professional status and any differences their class and race might produce. In none of the other consultations does a patient take a provider to task about a medical topic and prevail. Yet this exchange is quite similar to Katherine's interactions with Prudence. Katherine, too, locates herself as a woman like Prudence and locates Prudence as a person of class like herself.

When the topic is the context of her patient's life, Katherine supports Prudence's perceptions. She explains that she and most of the women she knows would not do well living in the atmosphere of Prudence's daily life. And, in doing so, she circulates an oppositional discourse about women, work, and the nuclear family. Claudia, too, circulates an alternative discourse about women, but for her the topic is sexuality. As she encourages Pat to masturbate, she also locates herself as a woman like Pat.

However, no sooner does she produce this solidarity and circulate this discourse than she switches to a discussion about the need for a heterosexual relationship in a woman's life and reproduces hegemonic understandings about women, heterosexuality, and the nuclear family. And here class and race may play a part. Perhaps looking for a good man is a different activity for a white, middle-class woman than it is for a poor, African American woman. If so, by not recognizing these differences, by not accepting Pat's description of her life as authoritative, Claudia both reinscribes her professional identity and undermines the solidarity she has produced with Pat. Although Katherine never speaks a hegemonic discourse about women, when she raises the topic of divorce for the fourth time and presses Prudence to accept her recommendation and when she pushes Prudence to do what is good for her even if her husband pouts, she too recirculates her professional identity. As the nurse practitioners move back and forth between these discursive positions, they make the pervasiveness of competing discourses visible.

Patients, too, locate themselves in ways that demonstrate the persistence of competing discourses. Although Pat consistently speaks from an oppositional position, challenging Claudia on both medical and social/biographical grounds, Prudence does not. She moves between discourses that reinscribe and those that dismantle dominant understandings about women, work, and the nuclear family. In addition, while both Prudence and Pat successfully resist the provider's definition of the situation, they are resisting opposing positions. Prudence withstands Katherine's oppositional treatment recommendations (divorce and therapy), and Pat counters Claudia's more hegemonic recommendation (that she seek a heterosexual relationship).

MEDICAL AND NURSING ENCOUNTERS: SUMMARY

Although there are differences between the two nursing encounters, they are more similar than different, especially when compared with the medical consultations. And these differences hold across presenting complaints coded as medical or marked as social psychological. The medical relationship is overwhelmingly characterized by a two-place logic—doctor/not doctor, man/not man, medical complaint/not medical complaint—that is entirely lacking in the nursing relationship. The nursing consultations are much more multilayered and complex. And this very complexity produces tensions that are entirely absent in the medical consultations.

There are other differences as well. Doctors consistently revivify their institutional authority, but nurses do not. The nursing encounter is more fluid, moving between positions that reinscribe and dismantle the asymmetry usually associated with the provider-patient relationship. Whereas both doctors marginalize the social/biographical, the nurse practitioners do not. Whereas all the providers transport social/ideological assumptions into their discussions, these assumptions are different in the medical and nursing encounters. Doctors insistently reinscribe dominant cultural assumptions about women, but the nurses do not. Both nurse practitioners circulate oppositional discourses about women and domestic arrangements. Even though Claudia speaks a hegemonic discourse about heterosexual relationships, she, like Katherine, also undermines other dominant understandings about gender.

These differences are reflected in both the decision-making process and the outcome. Although patients resist in each consultation, they are never successful with doctors but usually are successful with nurses. Whereas doctors stick to their definition of the situation despite consistent resistance from patients, nurses do not. In the end Katherine and Claudia respond to the their patients' resistance in the same way. They regroup, suggest an alternative, and push for a compromise, which they obtain.

These differences have an impact on the way health care is delivered. Wendy struggles with Doctor Aster about the cause of her presenting complaint—the conflict, or lack of conflict, between her domestic responsibilities and her labor-force participation. And Muriel struggles with Doctor Johnson about how appropriate it is for an older, recently widowed woman to be sexually active. The patients' complaints are located differently (social psychological and medical); however, the outcomes are the same. Both women lose their struggles; providers and patients agree on treatment recommendations; and patients leave the encounters with less than they came for. Wendy leaves without accurate information about birth control or a prescription for contraceptives. And Muriel leaves lacking essential information about the difference between a sexually transmitted infection and a venereal disease and without having reached an agreement about how her man friend should be treated.

Even though the struggles take place in a social register and circulate social/ideological assumptions about women, they are about a medical topic—diagnosis. The medical task is to identify the specific etiology of the presenting complaint.

Given the two-place logic so characteristic of the medical relationship, the social/biographical context is of little significance in reaching a diagnosis. It does not matter how Wendy feels about why she hyperventilated or how Muriel feels about her sexual behavior.

Moreover, once the diagnosis is made, it shapes the way health care is delivered as well as the treatment recommendation. Topics defined as marginal are left unaddressed.

In each nursing encounter, by contrast, the social/biographical and the medical interpenetrate each other, providing a richer account of the patient's life and its relationship to her presenting complaint. Again, even though the complaints are located differently (medical or social psychological), the outcomes are the same. There are no struggles about the causes of the presenting complaint or the diagnosis. Instead, in both encounters the struggles that take place in a social/ideological voice are about the way to treat problems once they are identified and agreed upon. Katherine and Prudence agree that Prudence's life is intolerable. They disagree about whether a divorce is the best way to solve the problem. And both Claudia and Pat agree that something needs to be done about Pat's social isolation. They disagree about whether a relationship with a man is the best solution.

The struggles in the nursing encounters, like those in the medical consultations, take place in a social register and circulate social/ideological assumptions about women (albeit different ones). But the topic, although medical, is different—treatment instead of diagnosis. Whereas in making a diagnosis the provider searches for a specific cause, recommending treatment is a different task. It is to figure out the course of action most likely to produce the patient's compliance. Nurse practitioners bring a flexibility to this task that is entirely lacking in doctors.

In both nursing encounters providers offer treatment recommendations—divorce and relationship. These recommendations are reached by talking about the context of patients' lives. Nevertheless each patient resists the provider's definition of the situation, and, at least initially, the patient prevails. Only after the providers modify their treatment recommendations in ways that honor what the patients have said about their lives are agreements reached. The social context of patients' lives counts in other ways as well. It influences the delivery of care. Patients talk broadly about their lives and the problems in them, and they leave the clinic having dealt with much more than their presenting complaints.

The medical and nursing encounters, then, are markedly different in the ways they include, or fail to include, the context of patients' lives, and this pattern is consistent with both complaints marked as social psychological and those coded as medical. In medical encounters information about patients' lives is discouraged and largely absent. In nursing consultations, by contrast, this information is abundant. These differences influence the way health care is delivered. There is little doubt that the context of patients' lives is important. In all probability as patients we would rather have providers, like the nurse practitioners, who encourage us to talk about our lives and pay attention to what we say.

However, while Katherine and Claudia encourage Prudence and Pat to speak about the social/biographical context of their lives, this speaking does not automatically remedy the problems frequently found to characterize the medical relationship. Quite the contrary. Nurse practitioners undermine their professional identities, but, like doctors, they also reproduce the characteristic asymmetry of the medical relationship. In addition, like doctors, they transport social/ideological assumptions into the medical discussion. But again there are important differences.

Whereas the doctors only recirculate hegemonic discourses about women and domestic arrangements, both Katherine and Claudia speak an alternative discourse. However, although Katherine speaks only in an oppositional voice, Claudia moves between discourses that undermine and recirculate hegemonic assumptions about women.

Teaching doctors to include the social biographical might increase the sensitivity with which they diagnose, treat, and deliver care. However, although a discourse of the social may be necessary, it is not sufficient. By itself, encouraging patients to speak about their lives does not even begin to address the pervasive ways that social/ideological discourses penetrate a presumably medical discussion or the reasons why these discourses are so different in the nursing and medical consultations. And these differences are significant.

In each encounter, provider and patient struggle over the definition of the situation and over whose interpretation of women's needs will be authoritative. Although in both medical and nursing encounters these struggles are social/ideological in nature, they perform different kinds of ideological work, which makes the production of knowledge visible. Doctors do not circulate oppositional discourses. They do not establish solidarity with women patients. And they do not dismantle their professional identity.

Instead, they insistently reinforce their identities as doctors and men. They speak the royal "we," locating themselves in a medical community. And, in addition, they position themselves in a community of men. Albeit subtly, Doctor Aster implies that men—doctor and husband—know what is best for women. He positions himself in a similar way when he explains that "most people" would agree that working at home and in the paid labor force is stressful. Although "most people" could refer to women as well as men, the unmarked category signals dominance and is usually gendered male.[11] In each case he reinscribes his identity and the asymmetrical nature of both medical and gender relationships.

Not only do doctors consistently reinscribe their location as doctors and men, but, notwithstanding patients' resistance, they also unrelentingly position women patients as others saturated with gender. As women they are overly emotional and dependent on men (whether doctors or husbands). As patients they are less than competent and prone to gab unnecessarily about the context of their lives.[12] Perhaps the two-place logic so common in the medical relationship plays a role here. If the doctor's position rests on the patients' location as other—not doctors, not men—then to treat them in any way except as other undermines this position. But whatever the explanation and despite the ways patients resist, doctors persistently reproduce hegemonic, gendered identities for women patients and thereby define them and limit their options while reinscribing their own gendered and professional identities.

Nurse practitioners produce knowledge about their gendered and professional identities and about women patients' proper place in medical and gender relationships quite differently. Although they certainly push to have their interpretations of patients' medical care and social lives considered authoritative, they also pay attention to patients' resistance. Without the two-place logic that characterizes the medical relationship, nurses can and do move back and forth between positions that reinscribe their professional identities and those that locate them as like their patients. They can and do reproduce their institutional authority and support the authority of patients' voices.

In addition, nurse practitioners do not position themselves as professionals by locating patients as gendered others. Even when Katherine and Prudence struggle, Katherine does not construct Prudence as other. While persistently speaking an alternative discourse, she supports Prudence whether Prudence is circulating hegemonic or alternative positions about women, work, and the nuclear family. Although the situation is not quite as clear cut with Claudia, most of the time she too supports Pat's authoritative voice and does so with both medical and social/biographical topics. And she speaks an oppositional discourse about women and sexuality almost as consistently as Katherine does.

Because nurse practitioners and patients are both women, gender is not as good a category on which to differentiate provider and patient as it is for doctors. Although Katherine and Claudia could make distinctions within this category—could produce patients as others by locating themselves as exceptional women, professional women, enlightened women, white women, women of class—for the most part they do not. But, perhaps even more important, neither Katherine nor Claudia positions her patient as gender-saturated. They present their patients as competent, not as overly emotional. And they encourage them to be their own person. While these persons are clearly gendered, gender alone is not sufficient to define them or their life options.

There is a price to pay for these differences. When Katherine and Claudia press to have their interpretation of Prudence's and Pat's needs considered authoritative, they are not successful. Katherine repeatedly recommends divorce, and Claudia strongly presses Pat to look for a relationship with a man. Each time these recommendations are made, both patients resist. Even in this situation, providers do not position patients as other. Instead, Katherine and Claudia bring to bear all the solidarity they have established and all the authority available to them. In so doing they move to reposition both themselves and the patients by reinscribing the institutional authority characteristic of the provider-patient relationship.

But the nurse practitioners do not prevail for at least two reasons.

Both of the patients persistently resist their definition of the situation, and both providers, at least on some occasions, have undermined the institutional authority associated with their professional status. In my opinion these factors set the stage for both Katherine and Claudia to abandon their initial recommendations and suggest alternative remedies.

Even though Prudence and Pat have resisted and prevailed, it would be a mistake to think that this outcome changes the structural location of provider and patient. While patients have much more leeway in these consultations than in the medical consultations, nurse practitioners still establish and maintain the parameters of what is, and is not, a legitimate topic for discussion. Although Prudence diagnoses herself and Pat tells Claudia how to treat her scab, in both cases nurse practitioners make the space for them to do so. They circulate their institutional authority or distance themselves from it, position patients as others or do not. These providers also push for an oppositional resolution to patients' problems. They interpret patients' needs and define the best way for them to live their lives, and they do so even after the patients successfully resist and they compromise. Both Katherine and Claudia suggest compromises. By doing so, although they pay attention to the context of the patients' lives, they still see their interpretation as authoritative. And in the end the providers' definitions, albeit compromises, prevail.

Several conclusions suggest themselves in these comparisons. First, once patients have been accorded some authority, it is not easy to take it back. Second, although I am sure there are other equally salient categories, gender plays a pivotal role in these encounters. It is either the basis for the production of solidarity or the foundation on which otherness is reinscribed. Third, there is an amazing persistence in the institutional patterns of interpretation that characterize the medical and the nursing encounters. From the opening moments, when the stage is set, through the ways solidarity is or is not established and competence is or is not produced, to the repetitive nature of the kinds of social/ideological struggles providers and patients engage in, the medical and nursing encounters provide different sites for the delivery of health care, the production of knowledge, and the negotiation of identities.

Finally, even though the medical and nursing encounters are quite different, it is far too simple to argue that nurses have added caring to curing, that they have added a discourse of the social to the medical discourse said to characterize the provider-patient relationship. Paying attention to the social/biographical context of patients' lives is important, but it seems much more reasonable to argue that neither caring as clinical practice nor a theoretical remedy is sufficient to address the problems just discussed. How better to address the nursing of wounds is the topic of the next chapter.

EIGHT

THE POLITICS OF LOCATION

I started this project after having been told that nurses do it better. They add caring to curing, and, in so doing, they provide better care for patients' physical complaints as well as their more social psychological wounds. For me this formulation is both tantalizing and problematic. As a feminist and a woman patient, the idea that nurse practitioners deliver health care in a more patient-centered way is appealing. But for several reasons it is also troubling.

First, nurses seem to be making an empty assertion. At the time I began this research, there were virtually no qualitative empirical data that provided a detailed description of what nurses actually did in examining rooms. Without this information, it is impossible to know whether caring or quality translate into a different kind of clinical practice and, if so, how.

Second, nurses are plugging into a liberal, reformist discourse that I find suspect. Reformers like Mishler (1984) argue that if doctors encourage patients to speak in a social/biographical voice, if they add the voice of the patient's lifeworld to the medical voice found to dominate doctor-patient consultations, they can minimize the asymmetry that characterizes these encounters and humanize them. Nursing locates itself in a similar manner. Not only do these presentations treat the medical and the social as two distinct realities, but they purge both of their structural context.

In a similar but slightly different manner, the way nursing positions itself professionally reproduces a liberal, reformist discourse that bases achievement on merit. If nurses add caring to curing, then they provide better health care and should have increased professional status. This merit-based conception of achievement cleanses it of all political considerations, while leaving intact the notion of an objective medical science. In addition, by basing their claim for professional status and their identities as providers on a system of care, they leave unchallenged the bifurcation of the medical and the social. Medicine remains the real stuff of clinical practice unsullied by social concerns. Nurse practitioners just add the gendered activity of caring.

By linking its claim to professional status to caring, nursing both obscures the workings of the dominant culture and unintentionally recirculates them. Because caring is coded as a gendered activity, if nurses, who are overwhelmingly women, care, and doctors, who are still predominantly men, do not, then medicine is reinscribed as gendered male, while caring and nursing are recirculated as gendered female. And in this society once a professional space is feminized, it is marginalized in both status and earning capacity.

The association of nursing with caring, then, runs the risk of reproducing the very gendered meanings and hierarchies many of us have resisted for years, reinforcing both a sexual division of labor and a secondary labor market. By participating in an us/them logic and locating the distinctive feature of those like us in caring, nurse practitioners inadvertently revivify the professional and gendered binaries they are attempting to subvert. From this perspective my previous criticism of a team approach to health care makes sense. In a team doctors are still the "top dogs" who do the "real stuff" of diagnosing and treating patients' medical problems, but nurses, as the new, somewhat elevated but still subordinate partners, now add the important but undervalued work of caring. Although these two providers may together perform interrelated but differently valued tasks and, in so doing, may improve the way health care is delivered, current economic, ideological, and institutional arrangements are also reproduced, albeit in somewhat modified form.

Given both the appeal of nurses' claim that they do it better and my concerns about that claim, my initial goals were to gather the missing empirical information, compare detailed descriptions of the ways doctors and nurse practitioners deliver care to women patients, and evaluate whether complaints marked as social psychological provide a more fertile site for a discourse of the social than do complaints coded as medical. In other words, I wanted to gather data on caring as clinical practice. These data speak quite clearly. Although there are important similarities in the ways nurse practitioners and doctors deliver health care, there are also significant differences.

I found that no matter how complaints were coded, the clinical practice of nurse practitioners certainly made space for patients' voices, but the clinical practice of doctors did not. However, while in nursing encounters patients were consistently encouraged to speak about the social/biographical context of their lives, speaking in this way neither was automatically liberating nor magically eliminated the asymmetry characteristic of the medical relationship. And although the clinical practice of doctors was different, it certainly did not lack a social discourse. In each consultation and with both kinds of complaints, a social/ideological discourse penetrated the presumed objectivity of health-care discussions and did so differently in the medical and nursing encounters.

Although, for me, these findings lessen neither the appeal of nurses' clinical practice nor my distaste for the ways doctors provide medical care, they leave important theoretical issues unaddressed. Clearly, the relationship between the medical and the social is more complex than it at first appears. This complexity is captured neither by the claim that nurses do it better nor by the argument that attention to the patient's lifeworld will remedy the troubles in the medical relationship.

To contruct theory from the strong and recurrent patterns in the five preceding chapters—patterns that characterized the ways the doctors and nurse practitioners delivered health care—in this chapter I return to Mishler's (1984) call for a discourse of the social and Silverman's (1987) and Waitzkin's (1983) different criticisms of it. Drawing on the empirical materials just presented, I consider how these theories both provide important analytic insights and leave equally significant areas unaddressed and, in their either/or theoretical formulation, unaddressable. Next, drawing on the insights of structural and discursive theories, I refashion the social/ideological. After I situate medicine and nursing in their historical, structural, and cultural locations and talk about situated knowledges, I discuss ways to understand the linkages among institutional sites, interpretive practices, and political processes.

By shifting to a somewhat different view of clinical practice and linking this view to an alternative understanding of how the ideological functions, I highlight both the constraints against and the opportunities for political struggles for social change. And, on this basis, I talk about alternative, and hopefully more potent, political strategies for nurse practitioners and suggest, in the Epilogue, some policies for remaking the American health-care system.

CARING AS A DISCOURSE OF THE SOCIAL REVISITED

When Mishler (1984) calls attention to the importance of the patient's lifeworld, he is speaking to troubles that are all too characteristic of the medical relationship.[1] These troubles are apparent in the cases just discussed. By sticking to the medical model and bifurcating the medical and the social, Doctors Aster and Johnson marginalize the social/biographical context. Without this social, contextual information, neither doctor adequately meets his patient's medical or social needs.

Katherine and Claudia, by contrast, do all that Mishler recommends. By not bifurcating the medical and the social and by expanding the medical model to include biographical information, both nurse practitioners more than adequately deal with Prudence's and Pat's needs—medical and social. However, although these practices may humanize the provider-patient relationship, they do not automatically liberate patients from the troubles in their lives or providers from the asymmetry characteristic of medical encounters. Instead, they generate struggles in a social/ideological register— struggles of a kind essentially lacking in medical encounters.

Mishler and others who dichotomize medicine and the lifeworld and declare that the social is found in the lifeworld direct attention away from the very issues that arise in these encounters. Although nurse practitioners encourage patients to talk about their lives and doctors do not, each provider transports a social/ideological discourse into presumably medical discussions, and these discourses are different. The doctors define Wendy's and Muriel's lives in ways that persistently recirculate dominant cultural assumptions about women. In so doing, they refigure themselves as men and medical experts. And although both nurse practitioners circulate alternative understandings about medical and gendered relationships, they also reinscribe hegemonic understandings. In fact, most of the struggles in the nursing encounters are organized by the tension between these opposing positions.

By limiting the social to the context of patients' lives, Mishler provides no analytic framework for addressing social/ideological discourses and, therefore, no way to deal with important differences between medical and nursing encounters. In addition, both nursing's claim that it offers a system of care and Mishler's call for a discourse of the social leave intact the assumption that medical discourse is objective. From this perspective there is no way to illuminate how a social/ideological discourse interpenetrates medical discussions and, therefore, no way to indicate how political provider-patient discussions are or how, in and through struggles that occur in a social/ideological register, health care is delivered, gendered and professional identities are negotiated, and cultural meanings are produced.

Silverman (1987) and Waitzkin (1983) each provide theoretical pieces that are missing in Mishler's analysis. Silverman is troubled by the distinction Mishler makes between medicine and the lifeworld. Rather than being oppositional, he describes them as voices that "interrupt and interpenetrate each other" (Silverman and Torode 1980:104). From this perspective providers do not speak solely in medical voices, and patients cannot speak the "truth" about their lives in authentic social voices and thereby liberate themselves.

This insight is important. It provides the analytic ground for exploring how knowledge is produced as social/biographical and how medical discourses interrupt each other. However, Silverman does not use this insight to show how these discourses interact. Instead, he shifts his analytic gaze away from the social and back to the medical. He claims that the distinction Mishler makes ignores "the place of medical discourse in modern societies and, indeed, the way it has entered our own account of ourselves" (Silverman 1987:198).

There is little doubt that the language of medicine has entered our accounts of ourselves and become part of our cultural understanding, but this description tells only part of the story. In all the consultations described, a social/ideological discourse is brought into the examining room, where it interrupts and interpenetrates a presumably medical discourse and does so differently in the medical and the nursing encounters.[2] Although Silverman's theoretical perspective certainly does not preclude an analysis of the social, it both directs attention away from the social and fails to specify its nature.

In this way, Silverman's position implicitly recirculates Mishler's coding of the social as the biographical and reproduces the medical and the social as distinct voices modified so that they can now be spoken by both doctors and patients. Here the binary medical/social—a binary Silverman tries to undermine—is reinscribed. But, even more important, because the nature of the social is not specified, there is no analytic framework from which to illuminate how social/ideological discourses are already incorporated into the discussion of both social/biographical and medical topics.

From this perspective, then, there is no way to address the patterns discussed in the preceding chapters. Whether providers and patients struggle about medical or social topics, their struggles are in a social/ideological register and are deeply political. There is also no way to account for why, by the end of each encounter, the provider's definition of the situation has prevailed.

By claiming that doctor and patient can speak in either medical or social voices and that these voices interrupt and interpenetrate each other, Silverman ignores what I am referring to as the politics of location. He ignores the place of medicine in larger structural arrangements as well as the institutional location of health care providers. From this perspective he has no way to analyze the relationship between voices. This position relies on a particular and not uncontested understanding of power. Drawing from Foucault (1981, 1979), he argues that power is neither something that can be possessed nor something that operates from above through constraint and repression. It is "capillary," circulating everywhere and in everyone. It operates in everyday social practices at the lowest rather than the topmost extremity of the social body and works as much through encouraging as repressing speech.

If, as Silverman claims, doctors and patients are "compelled to speak to one another in a common language around which a field of power forms to govern them both" (Arney and Bergen 1983, quoted in Silverman 1987:198), then medical domination no longer provides an appropriate model for understanding either the provider-patient relationship or challenges to it. It follows that neither medical providers nor social scientists can engineer new forms of practice. Change cannot come from above. It can come only from practical struggles. Silverman concludes by quoting Foucault: "the problem is one for the subject who acts" (1981:12–13, quoted in Silverman 1987:203).

Based on the cases just discussed, it certainly seems that power can work as much through encouraging as through repressing speech and that the provider-patient relationship is a site for struggle. Although Silverman makes this point, he does not take full advantage of it. His point provides a theoretical justification for examining the social/ideological struggles between providers and patients—struggles that clearly do not disappear if providers are encouraged to talk about the context of patients' lives. But to examine these struggles is to raise issues that are hard to deal with from Silverman's theoretical perspective.

If a social/ideological discourse provides a site for reinscribing or resisting hegemonic discourses—a site for struggle—does one have to reject any notion of medical domination and, instead, accept a shared capacity for action (subjects who act) and total reliance on a conception of power as productive? From Silverman's perspective the answer to this question is a resounding yes. However, it is hard to reconcile his position on medical domination, his conception of the subject, and his notion of power with the consultations just described.

If one discounts the way nurse practitioners open and close the discussions, ask most of the questions, and establish most of the topics, then power at least the power to speak dominant or alternative discourses—seems to circulate everywhere and in everyone. But this look is deceptive. Although in the first nursing consultation Prudence is caught between hegemonic and alternative discourses about women, Katherine is not. She consistently pushes oppositional understandings. And while Prudence resists and, on occasion, is successful, in the end Katherine's oppositional position prevails.

In the other nursing encounter the nurse practitioner, not the patient, is caught between dominant and oppositional discourses.

And although Pat accepts Claudia's oppositional recommendations, she struggles against the hegemonic one. Again, although the patient resists and is, on occasion, successful, in the end Claudia's hegemonic position prevails. Are nurse practitioners, then, the subjects who act, and, if so, how would Silverman account for what looks like medical domination?

If one looks at the doctor-patient consultations in terms of a shared capacity for action, the notion of power as productive is even harder to understand. Throughout the medical encounters Doctors Aster and Johnson reinscribe one version of reality. They foreground the traditional nuclear family—a woman who is defined by her domestic responsibilities or her state-sanctioned heterosexual relationship, and men, whether husbands or doctors, who know what is best for her. Although each patient struggles against the doctor's definition of the situation, neither is successful, not even once. The doctor's representation of the dominant order consistently prevails. If this is not medical domination, is the domination produced by a patient (subject) through her failure to struggle sufficiently?

In all the cases discussed, despite patients' persistent resistance, providers prevail, and the asymmetry of the medical relationship is recirculated. Although providers and patients may share a common language, a field of power does not seem to form to govern them both. Quite the contrary. Something very much like medical domination appears to be operating. Yet, from Silverman's Foucauldian position, questions about institutional authority, about domination and subordination cannot be posed, let alone adequately answered. For reasons such as these Fraser (1989) argues that a conception of power as productive, unavoidable, and, therefore, normatively neutral is problematic because, from this perspective, it is neither possible nor desirable to specify "who is dominating or subjugating whom and who is resisting or submitting to whom" (29).

The comparisons of the doctor-patient and nurse practitioner–patient consultations raise two additional questions that are neither addressed by nor addressable from Silverman's Foucauldian perspective. First, if doctors and nurse practitioners persistently put forth their definition of the situation and if, in the end, that definition prevails, how do we account for the differences between them or justify a preference for, or a commitment to, one side as opposed to another? Again, this is a question that Fraser (1989:283–286) raises. Although for her such justification and commitment are desirable, she points out that from a Foucauldian perspective they are not possible. For Foucault, normative neutrality allows arguments neither about power nor about morality. As a feminist Fraser finds normative neutrality disturbing, as do I. And as a theorist she points out that Foucault's position is particularly troubling because his notion of resistance already implies such a normative standard.

Second, if providers and patients are engaged in practical struggles, where does their power come from? Because Silverman is relying on a Foucauldian understanding, neither power nor resistance can be an expression of some preexisting structural or symbolic order. With power theoretically defined as productive, there is no conception of society. Yet, without a conception of society, it is impossible to assess how strong the power is, how strong the resistance is, or the changing balance between them (Hall 1986). From this perspective, then, there is no principled way to explain the differences in the medical and nursing encounters, no way to explain why doctors incessantly reinscribe hegemonic gendered and professional relationships but nurse practitioners do not.

Here is where structural criticism confronts Foucauldian analysis. From a structural perspective it is not difficult to locate which groups have power or why they wield it as they do. Nor is it difficult to justify a preference for one side over the other. While Waitzkin (1983), for example, does not explicitly talk about the social as the context of patients' lives, he does argue that medical discourse does not exist in a vacuum. It is deeply ideological and political, reflecting and reinforcing broader social relations. When patients talk about the trouble in their lives during medical consultations, doctors have an opportunity to do ideological work. Using the symbolic trappings of scientific medicine, they can encourage patients' consent to behaviors that are consistent with hegemonic or oppositional expectations and, in so doing, reproduce or undermine material conditions, especially economic conditions. If doctors analyze the social roots of suffering, if they avoid medicalizing nonmedical problems, and if they stimulate patients to become actively engaged in resistance, then they can become socially conscious agents of change.

Waitzkin, like Silverman and Mishler, seems to point us in the right direction, albeit a different one. He provides a notion of power as other than productive, links it to both a conception of society and the institution of medicine, and implies that whether the topic is medical or social the ideological work done during medical encounters reflects and reinforces larger structural arrangements. In the consultations described here it seems quite apparent that ideological work is being done and that this work recirculates cultural assumptions about professional and gendered relationships. Yet doctor and nurse practitioner do this work differently, usually circulating opposing cultural discourses. And from Waitzkin's theoretical position these differences are again hard to reconcile.

At the heart of his argument is the Marxist assumption that institutions reflect and reinforce material conditions and that individual agents can peel away their false consciousness. At one and the same time, Waitzkin relies on these assumptions and turns them on their head to argue that doctors can become revolutionary actors who see reality and use their institutional authority to inspire resistance. Doctors, whose power reflects and reinforces their location in broader social relations, can capitalize on their location and transform patients into revolutionary actors by encouraging them to take actions that challenge the structural conditions restraining them.

Although Waitzkin is certainly providing a politics of location, I nevertheless have trouble with this formulation. It seems internally contradictory. If doctors are positioned in institutions that reflect and reinforce their location in society, then they are not the oppressed, who are the typical revolutionary actors in a Marxist scheme. In addition, Waitzkin's reliance on a Marxist analysis and, therefore, on economic conditions is not helpful in understanding the consultations just discussed.

It is fairly easy to see how Doctors Aster and Johnson function as agents of social control. They consistently guide Wendy and Muriel toward behavior that reflects and reinforces hegemonic understandings about the relationship between doctors and patients and men and women and, in so doing, support dominant structural and economic arrangements. It is much more difficult to see how they can simultaneously become agents for social change, encouraging Wendy and Muriel to become revolutionary social actors engaged in organized political activity. There is nothing the slightest bit revolutionary about the ideological work that is done in these interactions. On both the nature of the medical relationship and the location of women in relation to work and the nuclear family or age and sexuality, both doctors insistently reaffirm neoconservative cultural meanings.

The nursing consultations are more complex. Katherine, who consistently speaks an oppositional discourse that encourages Prudence to resist the oppressive conditions in her life, could be seen as a revolutionary actor—an agent for social change. But, as she pushes for change, she also recirculates the institutional authority associated with her professional status. Although this sounds much like the role that Waitzkin imagines, it is only marginally successful. Using all the resources at her disposal, Katherine is unable to convince Prudence that she should get a divorce or that she and her husband should go into therapy. Although her compromise is oppositional, running, talking with friends, and changing jobs is far from revolutionary.

Claudia looks much less like the revolutionary provider Waitzkin is calling for. She, like Katherine, speaks an oppositional discourse and, on occasion, recirculates the institutional authority associated with her professional status. However, unlike Katherine, Claudia speaks about women in both alternative and dominant voices. Although encouraging Pat to masturbate is certainly not part of the dominant discourse about women and sexuality, the search for a good man and a heterosexual relationship is.

Waitzkin provides many of the pieces that are missing in the other theoretical formulations. He directs attention to the way medicine is located in society. The social is, for him, more than the biographical. It is a site for subversive social/ideological work, and the symbolic trappings of scientific medicine play an important role in doing that work. Nevertheless, he maintains the distinction between the social, defined as the social/ideological, and the medical. In so doing he preserves the notion that doctors can be objective medical experts. However, they can also become revolutionaries who guide their patients to mobilize and take political actions. Here, power flows in one direction only—from the provider to the patient. In the name of revolutionary social change, the institutional

authority characteristically associated with providers is both legiti-
mated and extended.

Waitzkin's dual focus on providers as agents of both social control and social change directs attention toward the ways they au-
thorize patients' resistance in society and away from the ways
patients exert their agency in medical encounters. From this perspective it is hard to understand the ideological struggles in the
consultations just discussed—struggles that shaped the delivery of
care, the production of knowledge, and the negotiation of identity.
And it is equally hard to account for the ways these struggles were
resolved. Since health-care providers are active and patients are passive, since power flows from provider to patient, how would Waitzkin account for the fact that when Prudence and Pat resist, the
nurse practitioners respond by reformulating their treatment recommendations?

In addition, if power reproduces material conditions, differences
in the medical and nursing encounters must be understood largely
in material—that is, economic—terms. In this formulation, doctors' and nurse practitioners' economic location accounts for the
disparate ways they enact the institutional authority associated with
their professional status and for the different ways they talk about
gender. But although this position may enable Katherine to dis-
cover the "truth" about society and as a political actor to both consistently support Prudence's resistance and speak that "truth" in an
authentic voice, Claudia's position is more ambiguous. She both
discovers and speaks the "truth" while encouraging Pat's resistance
and remains in a state of false consciousness while pushing for Pat's
compliance to hegemonic assumptions. Does this mean that Katherine and Claudia are located differently in the economic arrangements of society? I interviewed both women and have no evidence
to support that conclusion. Furthermore, even if Katherine is more
economically marginal than Claudia and is, therefore, more often
an agent of social change, why does Waitzkin present providers
(doctors) but not patients as revolutionary actors? Providers, especially doctors, are not usually economically marginal, but many patients, particularly women patients, are.

While Silverman's and Waitzkin's positions seem contradictory,
taken together and augmented they have the potential to loosen the

ideological from its fixed association with a material base while demonstrating that the delivery of care, the production of knowledge, and the negotiation of identity are contested processes that take place in dynamic and socially situated ways. And, in so doing, they can be used to support a reformulation of the politics of location.

RESHAPING THE SOCIAL/IDEOLOGICAL

Mishler directs us to the importance of the social but, for him, it is limited to the biographical. Although Silverman fails to specify the social and quickly moves away from it, he lays out a fully discursive position in which the world, reality, social practice *is* language. There is nothing else of any significance, no contradictory force, no political inflection. Waitzkin, by contrast, takes us straight to a politics and a strategy that tightly link the social/ideological to the material. In these theoretical positions the gap between a fairly rigid structural determinacy and a discursive position, which is in danger of losing its reference to material and historical conditions, seems too great to bridge. But others are working to refashion these either/or perspectives. For them the openness of postmodern theory is attractive, as is the notion that meaning is discursively constituted. But, although not easily accomplished, these ideological, cultural, and discursive practices must be connected to a field of material relations.

To make this connection Hall (1986), for example, repositions theorizing as an open horizon, not a series of closed paradigms. Even though Hall describes himself as operating within "the discursive limits of a Marxist position" (Grossberg 1986:58), he locates himself as post-Marxist and poststructuralist. He recognizes the need both to move beyond orthodox Marxism and to incorporate the insights of poststructuralism to formulate a theory of ideological struggle.[3] To make these linkages Hall refashions the distinction between "the real" and "the false" (Hall 1986:38) and redefines ideology in ways that are helpful in extending the analysis of the provider-patient relations just discussed.

For him, ideology is neither a mystifying "trick" nor a state of false consciousness. The social relations in which people exist are the "real relations" (Hall 1986:38). Our ideological categories position us, allowing us to grasp "an aspect of social process in thought, . . . to represent to ourselves and to others how the system works, why it functions as it does" (39). Hall explains that these inscriptions make a material difference. Because how we act in the world depends on our definition of the situation, their effects are real. Here, Hall makes clear that language plays an important role in loosening economic determinacy from its position over ideology. "Language is the medium *par excellence* through which things are 'represented' in thought and thus the medium in which ideology is generated and transformed. But in language the same social relations can be *differently* represented and construed . . . because language by its nature is not fixed in a one-to-one relation to its referent but is 'multi-referential': It can construct different meaning around what is apparently the same social relations or phenomenon" (36).

Moreover, drawing on the insights of Volosinov (1973) and Gramsci (1971), Hall suggests that economic relations cannot prescribe a single, fixed, and unalterable way of conceptualizing the relations in which people exist. Their existence "can be 'expressed' within different ideological discourses" (38). If there is not a single referent, a fixed ideological meaning, then the potential for struggle is ever-present, and ideology is the terrain for this struggle—a terrain for "'intersecting agents' and the 'intersecting of differently oriented social interest'" (Volosinov 1973:23, quoted in Hall 1986:40). The attention to language and the notions that it is both identity-producing and multireferential take us from an abstract theory of ideology to a more concrete analysis of how meanings are accomplished (Gramsci 1971, referred to in Hall 1986:40). It does not, however, suggest that discourses appear spontaneously, combine, and recombine with each other in a free-floating manner unrestrained by anything other than discursive elements themselves.

The ways Hall positions discourse within a field of material relations and points us toward an empirical analysis of how meaning is accomplished provide an insightful way of analyzing the provider-patient encounters discussed earlier. Doctor Aster and Wendy, Katherine and Prudence, and Prudence with herself struggle about the definition of women, work, and the nuclear family. Doctor

Johnson and Muriel, Claudia and Pat, and Claudia with herself struggle similarly but about the definition of women, age, sexuality, and heterosexuality. Each contest is on an ideological terrain. In each, ideas about men and women as well as about professional and gendered relations are recirculated, undermined, and, sometimes, transformed.

Although there is no apparent single, fixed economic referent for these struggles, neither can they be explained as just the outcome of free-floating discursive operations. Instead, we see in the nursing, but not the medical, consultations a process of ideological struggle—a war of positions—that articulates, deconstructs, or reconstructs particular sets of social relations and political positions. Although these relations do not arise in a one-to-one relationship with economic conditions, they may very well reflect these conditions and more. They reflect how the terrain has been structured and mapped out historically as well as the struggle to detach certain gendered and professional concepts and, in so doing, to undermine the givenness of a particular historical terrain—to undermine the hegemonic power the prior position functions to secure.

Nurse practitioners, although not necessarily speaking the "truth" about society, turn texts about gendered and professional relations upside down and furnish different meanings both about women's experiences and about professional relationships. They provide alternative ideological categories within which the women who are nurse practitioners and their patients can locate themselves, can represent to themselves and others how the system works, why it functions as it does. They do so by positioning themselves and their patients in another language, drawing them into another historical bloc (compare Grossberg 1986:54–55)—the social movement called feminism. Here we have another kind of politics of location—a politics that is both situated and politically inflected. Although not automatically liberatory, this politics undoubtedly makes a difference in the way health care is delivered and knowledge is produced.

However, from this perspective there is no similar way for nurse practitioners to locate the caring on which they base their claims for professional autonomy. When the professional skill and specialized knowledge on which their claim to professional autonomy are coded as caring, there is no other historical bloc, no social movement, no political inflection, no terrain on which to struggle, and, therefore, no war of position or politics of location. Caring, whether in the home or in the workplace, is firmly located as gendered and, as such, is marginalized and devalued.

Hall's analytic gaze is broadly focused on ideology, on discursive cultural struggles. He directs our attention to the intersecting of differently oriented social interests and to the multiaccentual and situated nature of discourses to provide for their political inflections. In so doing he gives us a way to understand how nurse practitioners can produce alternative meanings—gendered and professional meanings—but are not equally successful in positioning themselves as autonomous professionals. These insights are important, but to flesh out a refashioned politics of location additional questions need to be addressed—questions about how particular institutions are located in society and why they function as they do as well as about the relationships between and across institutional sites. Situated knowledges, social alignments, and institutional patterns of interpretation are helpful here.

SITUATED STRUGGLES AND SITUATED KNOWLEDGES

Harding (1991) and Haraway (1991), although not specifically addressing ideology, talk about situated knowledges both to correct what they depict as partial and distorted versions of traditional analyses and to provide an account of how power is associated with the production of knowledge. Their criticism is directed equally at the notion of a disembodied objectivity—a gaze from nowhere (Harding 1991)—and rival claims, which they read as knowledge from everywhere. They similarly criticize positions that argue that power flows in a top-down fashion from somewhere or is produced everywhere. Instead, using the metaphor of vision, Haraway (1991) calls for an insistent embodiment in which objectivity is an active perceptual system and knowledge seeking and knowledge making are socially situated practices. Taken together they are calling for a strong concept of reflexivity in which neither the doing of research nor the production of meaning can be separated from their cultural, social, and historical locations and both are of necessity pluralistic.

Rouse adds to the concept that power/knowledge is socially situated and of necessity pluralistic the notion that it "is always mediated by a 'social alignment'" (1991:659). Drawing on Wartenburg (1990), he explains that a "relationship between two agents is a *power* relationship only because and to the extent that other agents will normally respond to the two agents in ways coherently aligned with the dominant agent's action" (659). Therefore, for Rouse and Wartenburg, social alignments implicate larger social structures in the "apparently local and specific exercises of power" (Rouse 1991: 659). Although it does not specifically address ideology, this formulation sounds much like Hall's (1986) intersecting agents and the intersection of differently oriented social interests. But although Hall specifically locates this process in a field of material relations, Rouse and Wartenburg do not.

Although Harding (1991) and Haraway (1991) are primarily discussing the research process and Rouse (1991) the doing of scientific research, much of what they are saying is directly applicable to the cases just discussed. In each case the power to produce knowledge does not flow directly from some preestablished institutional source or agent. But neither is the delivery of health care based on some kind of disembodied, objective language game. To understand the active perceptual process through which research is produced, Harding and Haraway call on researchers to gaze back to the particularities of their socially situated research projects and locate themselves in them. If we borrow this concept to gaze back and locate doctors and nurse practitioners, it is clear that the institutions of medicine and nursing were constituted historically as gendered professions.

In the nineteenth century, doctors tied by race, class, and gender to other powerful men in foundations and government gained a state-supported monopoly to practice medicine. To achieve this end, they competed against other providers who were less interventionist and more involved with patients in the total contexts of their lives (Riessman 1983). The eventual victory of the medical profession—its consolidation of cultural authority and a professional monopoly—was more a social and political victory than a medical one.

Nursing has no similar history. It evolved in the context of a medical monopoly and as a women's occupation that relied on a gendered skill understood as natural—caring—and a gendered relationship to doctors accepted as given—subordinate. As women, nurses historically had few ties to the powerful in society, and, although united by gender from its inception, nursing was stratified by class, race, and, later, by educational status. This history leaves nursing without the political clout and internal cohesion of the medical profession,[4] and it places nurses in a different relationship economically. The medical profession gains from its location in a capitalist economy as doctors practice predominantly in a fee-for-service system. Nurses rarely practice autonomously, rarely gain economically. They are usually salaried employees—a position doctors encourage and hospitals and insurance companies reinforce.

In these histories the ideology of gender difference is reinscribed, caring is represented as a natural quality of women, and reality is bifurcated into separate but unequal spheres. Doctors and nurses are positioned in a gender hierarchy and a sexual division of labor. They are identified as social actors and members of gendered and stratified professional groups. Each group is represented as having a different relationship to the system of knowledge called medicine and to its patients. These depictions continue today in much the same way and are reproduced in what Fraser (1989) calls "institutional patterns of interpretation."[5]

This concept repositions theoretical discussions and makes them concrete in ways I find especially helpful. For Fraser, as for Hall, "the social is by definition a terrain of contestation. It is the space in which conflicts over rival interpretations of people's needs are played out" (Fraser 1989:157). In this Gramsci-like formulation, "struggles over cultural meanings and social identities are struggles for cultural hegemony" (6). But instead of focusing on the level of cultural discourse, as Hall does, Fraser examines the production of situated knowledges (Harding 1991, Haraway 1991), the production of institutionalized patterns of interpretation.

Fraser discusses how in a specific institutional site—the social-welfare system—and through discursive struggles, social reality is made and unmade. The institution of social welfare, like the institutions of medicine and nursing, does more than provide material aid or deliver care. In these sites "multiple axes of power, . . . crosscutting lines of stratification . . . and a complex process of group formation" (Fraser 1989:10) are constructed and deconstructed. Social-welfare clients and, by implication, patients play an active part in this process. They resist, contest, and sometimes disrupt dominant social practices.

But although social reality is made and unmade through institutional patterns of interpretation, the social-welfare apparatus, for Fraser, is just one institutional site among many. Here, like Rouse (1991) and Wartenburg (1990), she is talking about the formation of social alignments. While these alignments offer opportunities to undermine power, to evade or resist it, to disconnect it from its supportive alignments, or to find counteralignments (Rouse 1991: 659), for Fraser, the production of knowledge is constrained as well as constituted in these alignments. Like Hall (1986), she analyzes how contests among rival discourses are multiaccentual. In them the various interests of the state, competing interpretations associated with oppositional social movements, social science experts, and neoconservatives intermingle, often polemically. By analyzing the struggles among these discourses in a specific institutional site and between institutional agents and their clients, she draws "a map of late capitalist social structure and political cultures" (Fraser 1989:10).

Like Fraser, I explore how women's needs are interpreted in institutional sites. I find, as she does, that needs are not just given. It matters who is doing the interpretation and what socially authorized discourses are available. But where Fraser looks at one institutional site, I compare two, both of which claim the delivery of health care as their central task. This comparison displays a somewhat different view of the ways competing interests intersect and, therefore, a somewhat different structural and cultural map. It suggests that some institutional sites are more oppositional than others; therefore, it also matters where—at what institutional location—these interpretations occur. Mapping the histories, practices, and politics of medicine and nursing allows a refashioned politics of location to emerge.

In the institution of medicine socially authorized discourses skewed in favor of doctors are consistently recirculated. While patients resist by speaking rival discourses, they do not disrupt dominant cultural meanings or social identities. Despite these struggles, doctors consistently locate themselves as men, as medical experts, and, at least on gender-related issues, as neoconservatives. They insistently position women as other, as subordinate both as patients and by gender.

In these struggles, while multiple axes of power may come together to position doctors and patients, there seem to be few cross-cutting lines of stratification and a rather simple us/them kind of group formation. Repeatedly, the private patriarchy of domestic relations, the public patriarchy (Brown 1981) of larger social systems like medicine, and dominant cultural discourses about medical and gendered relationships are reinscribed. By drawing an interpretive map on the basis of these interactions, one could easily conclude that over time, in the institution of medicine, and through institutional interactions, hegemonic systems of interpretation are stabilized and reproduced.[6] But if one looks at the nursing encounters, this conclusion is not so easily drawn.

Nurse practitioners speak socially authorized discourses that recirculate their professional status and rival discourses that locate them as women of a certain age, class, and race who share some common experiences with their women patients. Each nurse practitioner speaks an oppositional discourse about women, and each provides the discursive space for patients to struggle and prevail. But the struggles are quite different. Katherine and Prudence struggle about an oppositional response to the troubles in Prudence's life, and Claudia and Pat struggle about the neoconservative proposition that Pat needs a man and a heterosexual relationship in her life. Each struggle produces the same response: the nurse practitioner reformulates her position, and a compromise is reached.

Here, providers and patients struggle over cultural meanings and social identities. In these struggles nurse practitioners move between their locations as women of a certain class, age, and race and as medical experts. And, in addition, while Katherine consistently speaks an oppositional discourse about women, Claudia moves between this position and one that circulates more hegemonic understandings. In each case, when patients resist and prevail, they undermine dominant cultural meanings about medical and gendered relationships. In these struggles, then, the interpretive map looks much more like the picture Fraser presents. Multiple axes of power, crosscutting lines of stratification, and a much more complex, multiaccentual process of group formation are apparent.

When Fraser talks about the multivalent and contested character of needs talk, she is talking about how social-welfare clients, by speaking rival discourses, not only represent different social realities but also display how these representations are "acts which intervene" (Fraser 1989:166). Patients, too, speak rival discourses and represent different social realities. Although these "acts" are undoubtedly important, in the medical consultations as compared with the nursing consultations it is easier to see how they are constrained and constituted by social alignments and much harder to understand how they intervene to either undermine supportive alignments or circulate counteralignments. By contrast, in the nursing encounters, because patients' rival discourses are at least partially successful, it is much easier to see them as successful interventions, as counterhegemonic acts.

For Fraser, resistive acts such as these are part of ongoing political battles and, by extension, part of what I am calling a refashioned politics of location. In these battles, although power may determine the outcome, smaller counterhegemonic "publics" nevertheless ferment contestation, only slowly and laboriously. This process is easier for me to see in the nursing than in the medical consultations. Medicine and nursing, with their different histories, provide distinctive opportunities for these resistive acts.

This same process is clearly visible in nurse practitioners' struggles for professional autonomy and in the way they represent the delivery of care. Although far from totally disrupting the more powerful social alignments that support the institution of medicine, these acts "intervene." They undermine the notion that medicine is the only game in town. And they join nurses with others who are calling for a more humanistic practice of medicine, forming counteralignments. Although the medical profession has the strongest voice in this struggle and nurses are continuously vulnerable to the charges that they are not "real" doctors and are practicing medicine without a license, they are, nevertheless, slowly and laboriously fermenting a challenge to the medical monopoly that doctors have held since the early twentieth century.

Given the location of nursing as a relative newcomer to the state-sanctioned practice of medicine and as a gendered profession historically seen as subordinate, nurse practitioners are struggling from the margins to crystalize a professional identity as autonomous providers, as other than doctors' handmaidens. Like oppositional social movements, like clients in social-welfare agencies or patients during medical and nursing consultations, they are engaged in struggles over cultural meanings and social identities. Here, because the struggles are about professional class formation and institution building, nurses are struggling from below to remake a social reality that the medical profession has a vested interest in perpetuating.

It is no wonder, then, that the medical profession responds by restating its own position with increased vigor and by undermining the position of nurse practitioners. With a health-care delivery system in crisis and an ongoing political discussion about reforming it, the opportunity to remake social alignments through public policy is all too real. But to be active players, nurse practitioners cannot claim to do what doctors do only better. Nor can they claim to be members of a health-care team or autonomous practitioners who just add an essential missing piece—caring—to the delivery of health care.[7] Caring or a more humanistic practice of medicine may be a necessary discourse, but it is not a sufficient one. To undermine the medical hegemony and engage productively in the policy-making process, nurse practitioners will have to press their point differently. Their struggle to provide a different kind of provider-patient relationship and to gain a secure professional footing must be renamed and its politics made explicit. The discourses to set these changes in motion are already in play.

Political discourses about the health-care system stress fairness (equality of access), cost containment, primary care, patient education, and lifestyle changes. At the same time, in consumer discourses, patients are pushing for a more egalitarian provider-patient relationship in which there is a more trustworthy sharing of information and in which patients have a larger voice in the decision-making process. To gain the attention of the state and of consumers nurse practitioners will have to position themselves in relation to these discourses. And this positioning should not be difficult for them. Historically the ways they have delivered care are consistent with both discourses.

Here, theory and practice come together, and again Fraser's (1989) insights are helpful. It could be argued that if all institutions' locations are culturally constructed and discursively interpreted, if all are rooted in specific interested locations, then all are equally compromised. Fraser disagrees. She claims that all interpretations are not equally compromised, and by extension neither are all institutional sites. She provides principled ways to choose among these sites and argues that these choices are politically important, and I agree. To make these choices she asks three questions that I both borrow and modify. How hierarchical or egalitarian are the relations? Do the institutions and practices conform to, rather than challenge, societal patterns? What institutions and practices are most likely to support the transformation of health care into a right for all?

The institution of nursing and the practices of nurse practitioners developed differently from the institution of medicine and the practices of physicians, and they continue to have a different relationship to the system of knowledge called medicine and to their patients. They are more egalitarian and less hierarchical; they more often challenge rather than conform to societal practices; and they have a history that supports health care as a right for all. Both the ways nurse practitioners deliver health care and the ways they produce knowledge and negotiate identities most closely approximate the ideals of democracy, equity, and fairness. On these grounds the potential for continued struggle exists.

The institution of nursing and the clinical practice of nurse practitioners provide important political sites. In examining rooms the ways nurse practitioners interpret women's needs is political. In the public arena their professional discourse should be equally political. It should position them and what they do in ways that both disrupt the supportive alignments that sustain medical and gendered hierarchies and offer opportunities to form potent counteralignments. A politics of location is refashioned in this coming together of the politics of public discourses and the politics of the institutional interpretation of women's needs.

EPILOGUE

MAKING HEALTH-CARE POLICY

In addition to providing distinctive sites for the delivery of health care, the production of knowledge, and the negotiation of gendered and professional identities, the institutions of medicine and nursing offer different possibilities for dealing with the current health-care crisis in the United States. Despite the recent growth of family medicine, the medical profession as a whole has a longstanding commitment to high-technology specialty care and a much poorer record with regard to primary and preventive care. With the graying of the population and the possibility of universal access to health care, the need for primary and preventive care will only increase. Even if doctors were the best professionals to meet this need, by some accounts it would take about fifty years to train enough primary-care physicians. However, this is just the kind of care that nurse practitioners routinely provide, and as we learned in the sixties, they are much more easily trained.

While people inside and outside of government agree that changes are needed in the current health-care delivery system, most of the discussion focuses on what the health-care package should include, how to finance it, and whether we can afford universal coverage at this time. In the current fiscal climate, policy makers debate whether a single-payer system, managed care, or some other arrangement would be better. Personally, I favor a single-payer system and fear that managed competition will create an insurance oligarchy. Managed competition, insurance reform, or any of the other suggested remedies will not guarantee universal access to health care, cannot produce the necessary cost savings, and will not provide the same quality of care for all. At best each of the financing plans suggested, except for a single-payer system, will reproduce a tiered mechanism for the delivery of care, one in which access and quality of care are closely linked to financial status.

Regardless of how health care is financed, there is a strong possibility of a turf war. Doctors argue that only they have the medical knowledge and technical skill to deliver care. Cost-conscious policymakers and doctors protecting their professional turf talk about a team approach, with physicians remaining in charge and nonphysician providers, physician extenders, doing much of the routine and dirty work while keeping the costs down. But nurse practitioners claim that studies have repeatedly found that they deliver primary care as well as, if not better than, family-practice doctors (see Shamansky 1985). This claim entitles them to a piece of the health-care pie. Many want to be autonomous caregivers with prescriptive privileges, the ability to hospitalize and treat patients, and equal access to insurance coverage.

While there are no easy solutions, the problem needs to be reframed. Neither a team approach to health care nor giving nurse practitioners the autonomous ability to do everything that doctors do is sufficient to deal with the troubles in our health-care system. A team approach relies on a distributive injustice that reproduces gendered and professional hierarchies and a secondary labor force. And fully autonomous paraprofessionals would duplicate, rather than extend, the available services.[1]

However, if we consider the political process from which the present health-care system developed, lessons from recent history, and the experiences of other industrialized nations, we can find other ways to increase cost effectiveness and to reconceptualize the health-care delivery system. Current discussions fail to differentiate the high-technology specialty care that has historically been the province of physicians from the primary and preventive care that is so much a part of the way nurse practitioners deliver health care. Instead, the medical and the nursing professions have an additive model. To provide the needed preventive services, medicine adds a new specialty, family medicine, or broadens the care provided with physician extenders. And nursing provides medical care while adding caring and attention to the social psychological context of patients' lives to curing.

This is a nonsystem. All doctors, regardless of specialty, can provide primary care, and most doctors, even family practitioners, can provide some specialty care. While family doctors and nurse practitioners compete to provide similar services, only nonphysician providers—nurse practitioners, physician's assistants, and alternative practitioners—have their ability to practice limited in any significant way. As a society we pay for this lack of organization in rising costs and inadequate services.

Like other industrialized nations we need two integrated levels of care. Nurse practitioners, physicians' assistants, chiropractors, and other alternative providers should offer a broad community- and home-based system of primary and preventive care. They should also act as gatekeepers to another level of specialty care. We know from our experiences in the sixties and seventies as well as from the experiences of many other countries that 70 to 80 percent of the problems patients bring to doctors' offices could be handled just as competently by well-trained nonphysician providers. These experiences have been verified in official government reports (Graduate Medical Education National Advisory Committee 1979, 1980). In addition, an article in the *New England Journal of Medicine* suggests that many people, about one-third of the population and especially those with chronic conditions, are turning to and are often most constructively helped by alternative practices (Eisenberg et al. 1993). We also know that these providers cost less to train, increase access to care, and offer services that both cost less and are cost-effective in other ways as well (Graduate Medical Education National Advisory Committee 1979, 1980).

Family-practice doctors should be free to participate in this primary level of care or to practice with other specialists. All primary-care providers should be autonomous—not under the supervision of others—free to prescribe, and fully qualified for reimbursement. But except for midwives, who should be able to accompany their patients to hospitals if the need arises, they should not have hospital privileges.[2] Primary care should be the gateway to specialty care, and those at both levels, while limited to their spheres of expertise, should cooperate and communicate with each other.

Because President Bill Clinton invited those of us thinking about these problems to share our thoughts with him, I did. In my letter I shared both a widely accepted view of the problems facing us and the potential benefits in reorganizing the health-care delivery system into two integrated systems of care. The common knowledge is that the Clinton administration received thousands of similar suggestions. Yet neither the presidential initiative nor the public participation were enough to displace the status quo.

Perhaps a full and open discussion of all the thinking about how to improve and pay for a more equitable, humane system of health care, using the model of the economic summit, would have changed the outcome. Instead, the meetings to discuss these vital issues were held behind closed doors, and we were presented with a fully formed plan. This plan, portrayed as midway between the single-payer system, which Canada has and which many liberal Democrats support, and the Republican plans, which claim that there is either no crisis or none that a little tinkering around the margins could not repair, was poorly understood and lacked popular support.

In my opinion, wide-ranging popular discussion is still needed. I am including the letter I wrote to the Clinton administration with just a little editing. It provides a fitting epilogue to the book and perhaps will facilitate further discussion of this important topic.

I suspect that my view of the problems facing us is little different from your own. We are the only Western industrial nation, except South Africa, without some form of national health insurance. We have thirty-five to thirty-seven million people who are uninsured, and millions more are underinsured. People who lose their jobs, lose their insurance. Even if they are still working, people who become critically ill can have their benefits slashed. And people who become chronically ill can be reclassified as uninsurable or have their illness declared an uninsured exemption. In many states even an adopted baby is declared an uninsured exemption. All of this happens in a country that spends more of its gross national product on health care than do the other industrial nations that have some form of national health insurance.

At the same time, the health care delivered in the United

States is among the best, if not the best, in the world. We contribute significantly to research and development and have been innovators in the development and use of sophisticated technologies and procedures. However, we do not place the same kind of emphasis on primary care. Our health dollars are disproportionally spent on technological fixes like neonatal intensive care and open-heart surgery rather than on routine screening and more mundane preventive and primary care. In addition we spend most of these dollars in the last days of life rather than throughout the lifespan. We allocate our resources in this way despite the evidence that primary and preventive care are both life-saving and cost-effective. For example, as Gleeson points out in an unpublished position paper, for each dollar spent on providing prenatal care for low-income women, $3.38 is saved on the care of low-birth-weight infants, and the outcome in both healthy babies and a healthy parent-child bond is often better.

In the current organization of health care the insurance industry and the fee-for-service delivery system have both contributed to the problem. They have fought against any kind of national health-care system and supported tertiary rather than primary care. They have been resistant to cost controls, even when seeming to comply.

All over the country insurance costs are skyrocketing while people—more and more people—are becoming disenchanted. They see their premiums being raised and their coverage cut. If they have potentially expensive medical conditions, they see themselves being discriminated against either in their ability to get coverage or in the cost and terms of the coverage available to them. Even today, when some kind of national plan seems almost inevitable and when the insurance industry is talking about the need to provide an "essential package" of health benefits to all Americans, they are talking only about changing their pricing policy. Instead of establishing costs by distinguishing good from bad risks—experience rating—they will now provide a basic package of insurance at one price for all consumers—community rating.

The insurance industry has not been the only gatekeeper

locking some out while providing quality care for others. They are joined by doctors, who can and do choose whether to be primary-care providers or specialists, where to practice, whom to serve, what procedures to perform, and what to charge. Most doctors in the United States today choose to specialize, clump in more affluent areas, serve primarily people who are insured, and charge what the market will tolerate. These decisions create a situation rife with potential abuses. The statistics on the performance of unnecessary procedures and the dollars spent on high-technology fixes rather than on prevention and primary care speak clearly. We have more specialists per capita than other Western industrial nations and, therefore, more specialty procedures, from tonsillectomies and hysterectomies to open-heart surgeries. And although some can choose from among several specialists and receive the best care money can provide, the geographic maldistribution of medical services leaves many others—whole communities—medically underserved. These people are left for the public sector to deal with—a sector struggling under growing pressures and increasingly unable to provide adequate care. And things are not much better in health-maintenance organizations, where costs have also soared, savings are not passed on to patients, and there is a financial incentive *not to provide costly care—to undertreat.*

Although these practices steadfastly protect the profit-making interest of the insurance industry, the medical profession, and the health-maintenance organizations, their consequences are clear to see. The current organization of health care leads to abuses, and it does so at the cost of the overall health of our population. The infant-mortality rate in the United States has risen again. We are now twenty-third in international rankings. And in life expectancy for men we are twentieth. These are shocking statistics, especially for a country that prides itself on having the best health-care system in the world.

These problems are deeply entrenched and certainly not amenable to an easy fix; however, the current organization of our health care system is neither a historic necessity nor immutable. It is instead the result of a kind of historical accident.

Early in the twentieth century, under the rubric of educational reform, allopathic physicians gained control over a plethora of other providers. In their struggle for control, they chose a path different from that of many other countries. Instead of institutionalizing two integrated levels of health care, we institutionalized one. Instead of having a broad base of primary-care doctors who refer to a smaller group of hospital-based specialty physicians, we have one kind of doctor—the highly trained specialists free to practice any kind of medicine anywhere they choose. And when in the depression of the 1930s these doctors and the hospitals they used were having trouble collecting their fees, we institutionalized an insurance system that from its inception put the interests of hospitals and doctors ahead of the interests of patients, ahead of the social good.

I suggest we rethink these historic accidents in light of our current problems. If we take our lessons from our more recent history, we have good evidence about the kinds of things that work. When in the late sixties and early seventies we rediscovered poverty and the associated inequities in health care, the federal government acted to finance the training of family-practice doctors as well as two new paraprofessionals—the nurse practitioner and the physician's assistant. They also financed the development of a system of community clinics staffed by these primary-care providers. There are at least two lessons to be drawn from this time, and they are valuable lessons.

First, community-based care works and is cost-effective. As Gleeson reports in an unpublished position paper, it keeps people healthy and out of the hospital, and it saves money. She cites a Canadian study comparing community-clinic patients with private-practice patients; the community-clinics' patients cost 13 percent less than the private patients and had 23 percent fewer hospital days. If we expand a system of community clinics to include associated home and alternative care, the benefits are even greater. For example, Gleeson claims it costs approximately $800 per day to provide in-home care for AIDS patients versus $3,000 per day for hospital care. Using a report from the Government Accounting Office she argues that 20 to

40 percent of the elderly currently in nursing homes would not be there if help were available in the home or in the community. If we offered home- and community-based prenatal care, we would save the millions of dollars spent on low-birth-weight babies. And many chronic problems are dealt with in the most cost-efficient manner by alternative practitioners.

Second, paraprofessionals provide high-quality, cost-effective care. Despite repeated findings that nonphysician providers are as competent as family-practice doctors and have better social psychological skills, a stronger orientation to education and prevention, and lower costs per patient, their ability to practice has consistently been limited. Neither the quality of their performance nor the cost savings and health benefits associated with the use of paraprofessionals and the availability of community-based clinics and home health care have been enough to save them from the competitive pressures of the AMA and the cost cutting of the Reagan/Bush years.

If we do not talk about more than health-care financing and reorganize our health-care system, the changes we make may face the same fate as those that were made in the late sixties and early seventies. They will run the risk of being whittled away again sometime in the future. I suggest that we implement and institutionalize a system of primary care that includes home care, community-based clinics, and a range of alternative practitioners. This system should be geographically well dispersed, as public health services are today. Perhaps the public-health system and this new system of primary care should be combined in one institutional framework. But, however organized, this system should be broad-based, offering a range of services for mental and physical problems, from medical care and prescription drugs to alternative care, vitamins, and herbal remedies. It should also include the kinds of care routinely excluded from most insurance coverage: mental-health services, dental procedures, eyeglasses, eye refractions, visual therapy, and hearing aids. And it should be oriented toward primary preventive care and universally available. Universal access to the health-care system should be through this primary level of care.

In addition to the health benefits associated with these changes there are several other advantages. By establishing universal access to the health-care system through an institutionalized level of primary care, we would finally do away with the inequities associated with the current system—a two-tier system that provides one kind of care for the poor and poorly insured and another for the rich or well insured. Moreover, a system that uses primary-care providers as gatekeepers allows for local implementation of national policy and places decision making in the most appropriate hands—medical rather than bureaucratic. It also makes the most efficient use of health-care providers. If universal access to specialty medical care was through referrals from community-based, primary-care clinics, we also would have institutionalized a universal cost-management procedure. Medical problems, routine preventive and well-person care, which could be effectively handled in low-cost, primary-care community clinics, would not be referred to high-cost specialty physicians. And these primary-care providers would have no financial incentive either to provide unnecessary treatments or to withhold necessary ones.

There are two additional benefits. First, educational loans could be paid back with community service; a newly established system of broad-based primary-care clinics and associated home-care programs would provide an ideal site for such service. Second, we would anticipate a problem and institutionalize its solution. If we achieve some kind of health-insurance package for the approximately sixty million people who have been uninsured or underinsured, the current health-care system will be swamped both by the tremendous influx of people and by the magnitude of their medical problems. The people most in need of medical care will be those who are marginalized or are locked out of the current system. Their medical problems will overwhelm the system. There are not enough physicians to meet this increased demand for services. It would take many years to train enough primary-care doctors to meet this need. And given the organization of the current system, even with cost-containment mechanisms, costs will continue to soar.

A broad-based system of community clinics and associated home health programs dispersed in communities throughout the United States and staffed by a wide range of primary-care providers, including nurse practitioners and alternative providers, could help ameliorate some of the problems in the current health-care system while offering potentially valuable benefits. It would increase access to care while controlling costs and through education and prevention would decrease the need for additional care. In the future it might even help us achieve universal health care.

NOTES

ONE   *Nurses Do It Better*

1. In the late sixties, in response to the rediscovery of poverty as a social issue, two new health-care providers came into being: the nurse practitioner and the physician's assistant. Both were intended as "physician extenders." For years the supply of physicians had been maintained at an artificially low level, guaranteeing physicians both status and profit. But with the discovery of poverty came the concomitant discovery that whole sections of the population and whole areas of the country were medically underserved. Physician extenders were intended to extend the doctor's reach and, in so doing, to provide primary care to many of the underserved. To become primary-care providers, nurse practitioners and physician's assistants received additional training in clinical practice. For physician's assistants this training was provided in medical schools; for nurse practitioners it was provided in nursing schools. Today most nurse practitioners have a master's degree and are clinically prepared in a variety of subspecialties.

2. In this book (Fisher 1986), I explore how women are encouraged to have some treatments but not others.

3. I discuss my rude awakening in the first chapter of Fisher (1986).

4. An article in the nursing literature points out that nursing is "reaffirmed as being crucial to society *only* in times of shortage and systematically devalued at other times" (Lynaugh and Fagin 1988:184). I emphasize *only* here to support and augment their point. In fact, my concern about the ways nursing has rested its claim to authority on caring, my criticism of a doctor-nurse team approach to health-care delivery, and my complaint about the way professionalism internally stratifies nursing are each rooted in this history. Although I am certainly not alone in these concerns, criticisms, and complaints, the ways I suggest ending nursing's historic roller-coaster ride are, as far as I know, new. I argue strongly for the need to institutionalize primary care through a broad system of community clinics and associated home health services staffed primarily by nonphysician clinicians, alternative health providers, and those primary-care doctors who wish to participate. Not only would institutionalizing this kind of primary care provide the greatest social good, but it might finally end the marginalization of nursing.

5. For all too many years nurses were unequivocally doctors' handmaidens (Melosh 1982). In the beginning they replaced the family as caregivers, and later they provided the caring doctors all too often did not offer. For so long as they remained in a subordinate position as handmaidens, the hostility between medicine and nursing was minimized. Whenever they challenged that position, a struggle

ensued; and in these struggles nursing usually lost. For example, in the 1920s, when nurses were hired by patients as private-duty caregivers, they were able to function as patients' advocates. From this position they could challenge the health-care delivered by physicians. This potential upset the balance between medicine and nursing, and a struggle soon produced a different situation in which the relative autonomy of private-duty nursing was first diminished and then lost (Reverby 1987). And again in the 1960s nurses pressed to change their subordinate status. This pressure produced a response—the team approach to the delivery of care—that many doctors, nurses, and nurse practitioners support (compare Roueché 1977).

However, for me and many others in the caring professions, the team approach both rests on faulty assumptions and reproduces the gendered and professional hierarchy of medicine and nursing. According to its rhetoric a team approach replaces subordination with a realignment of roles based on the collaboration and colleagueship of professionals who have diverse but complementary skills. Combining these skills provides a better basis for medical decision making than the subordination model and, thus, offers better patient care. But when what differentiates nursing from medical skills is nurturing, caring, supporting, comforting, counseling, or even providing primary and preventive care and when these skills and the clinical practices that flow from them are devalued in the health-care system and in society, how can there be equity of any kind? Perhaps the clearest way this lack of equity is expressed is in the composition of professional boards. While doctors sit on nursing boards, the reverse is not true. Moreover, when doctors are primarily in fee-for-service practice and nurses are usually salaried employees, there are not only status differences but different economic interests. Even when doctors, nurses, and nurse practitioners are employed in similar situations—prepayment plans—their economic interests are often quite different. Nurses do not usually receive bonuses, but doctors usually do (Smoyak 1977). The more highly skilled the nurse is, the more damaging a team approach is. For nurse practitioners, it cools out a much more radical approach by undercutting the potential for groups of professionals with overlapping skills to compete.

6. Much of the material in the next three subsections of this chapter have already been published elsewhere (Fisher 1991, 1993).

7. Although others also make this point, I found the history provided by Reverby to be the most compelling. I rely strongly on it in this discussion.

8. This reliance on professionalism has a potentially devastating consequence for nurse practitioners. It establishes a hierarchy based on education and credentials—a hierarchy that all too often reproduces stratifications based on class and race—and it divides one kind of nurse from another, undermining the cohesion necessary for successful political action.

9. At first glance their argument seems quite similar to the position ethnomethodologists like Cicourel (1964) and Mehan and Wood (1975) have taken. However, current feminist theorizing is both more politically motivated and more oriented to an epistemological critique of the production of meaning.

10. Do we call these insurance or payment privileges? This very question suggests the kinds of structural constraints on nursing practice.

11. Although in one setting or another all but one of the nurse practitioners (the only male practitioner) are still delivering care, as of this writing only one is in the same setting. Five of the six remaining in practice changed jobs in an attempt to find a more supportive institutional setting, good medical backup, better pay, a more specialized clinical practice, or a situation that did not drain them in quite the same way (or a combination of these requirements). Perhaps these changes indicate a high level of burnout, which marks the frustrating conditions in which most nurse practitioners provide care. They work in settings where they see the relationship between poverty and illness everyday—a relationship they can do little to alleviate. They are overworked, underpaid, and, perhaps most important, attacked rather than appreciated by the doctors who should be their colleagues.

12. Although I cannot specify how their political commitments affected their clinical practice, my intuition is that a shared political stance was a significant factor. This intuition raises two other questions that I do not currently have the information to address. First, times have changed, and it is my impression that many women who identify themselves as feminists or as having left-of-center politics (or both) are choosing medicine instead of nursing. If I were to gather the same kind of qualitative empirical data about the clinical practice of these doctors, would the interactions look more like those of the nurse practitioners in this study or of the doctors? Or would they be more of a hybrid? Second, while nursing today is 97 percent women, if the kinds of women choosing nursing are changing and if men are becoming nurses in increasing numbers, has their political stance changed and, perhaps more important, will the clinical practice of these nurses change so that it looks more like the medical than the nursing practices I document here? Or will it, too, become some kind of hybrid? In other words, the practices I report on here and the conclusions I draw are historically grounded. As the social context changes, the ways that the "pervasive axes of inequality along lines of class, gender, race, ethnicity and age" (Fraser 1989:165) combine and the ways that the political responses to these factors change offer fresh opportunities for empirical research.

13. In the end, my interest in women and the construction of their identity shaped my focus, and I analyzed only the interactions with women patients.

14. I could not show either the details or the developmental nature of the production of meaning in any other way.

15. In this setting I did not observe an individual practitioner for a whole clinical session. Instead, I followed practitioners into the examining room outfitted with a video camera when they were going to be examining a woman patient. This is the only setting in which I have been able to both videotape and audiotape provider-patient interactions.

16. Although the primary-care doctors were residents and the nurse practitioners were more experienced, this difference did not affect the intended research. I was not evaluating primarily the way they provided medical care.

17. Every time I discuss this work doctors in the audience are upset. They tell me that I am being unfair. The doctors I am presenting are atypically bad and the nurse practitioners atypically good. Yet when I talk to other groups—the public more generally, women's groups, academics, students, public-health people, and nurses —what I am describing largely rings true. After years in examining rooms

watching doctors deliver health-care, this is my position as well. The specifics vary; nevertheless, the asymmetry, lack of attention to context, and support for the nuclear family and women's place in it are far from being atypical. Unfortunately, many researchers (Davis 1988, Waitzkin 1983, Mishler 1984), including myself (Fisher 1986, Fisher and Todd 1986), have found that they are all too common.

When women doctors are in the audience, especially those who identify as feminists, the problems they experience with my presentation are exacerbated. For obvious reasons they want to believe that women doctors, especially feminist women, do it differently. Their criticism of my presentation, although understandable, sidesteps what we already know and misses the point of this analysis. It is widely acknowledged that medical school and residency training are powerful socializing experiences. We know that even with the influx of women medical students the institution of medicine remains a largely male preserve. Men predominate in positions of authority. The dominant ideologies—fighting disease, controlling patients (assuring compliance), and insisting on hierarchy—are frequently associated with maleness. Historically, although women medical students and residents could fight for change, to make it through the system they largely had to play the male game and play it better than their male counterparts.

Has this situation changed? That is an empirical question without a ready answer. Certainly in the late seventies and early eighties, when I gathered data in a medical setting in the Southeast, women were in the minority, and their political and social attitudes were much like those of their male colleagues. At that time I found little difference in the way they and their male counterparts dealt with patients. Perhaps today there is a critical mass of women, especially women who identify as feminists or have other strong political commitments (also see note 12), who can join with other groups who have historically been marginalized and fight to change the system. Perhaps they will change the ideology of clinical practice, or, at the least, perhaps as individual practitioners they will deal with patients differently, but this remains an open empirical question—a question that may organize my next research project.

18. A word to readers who skip or postpone the reading of Chapter Two. The discussions of feminist theory and of the histories of the medical and nursing professions are helpful but not absolutely essential for understanding the conclusions in Chapter Eight and the policy recommendations in the Epilogue. After reading Chapter Seven, you might want to return to Chapter Two or use it as a resource when reading Chapter Eight.

TWO　*Situated Knowledges*

1. I am indebted to Donna Haraway (1991) and Sandra Harding (1991) both for the concept of situated knowledges and for many of the ideas discussed in this chapter.

2. Although he talks only about doctors, this is the position Waitzkin (1983) takes.

3. In early works written from an ethnomethodological perspective, Mehan lays out this perspective theoretically (Mehan and Wood 1975) and empirically (Mehan 1979). Although he is talking about education and not medicine, in many ways the position he takes is the forerunner of the later, more radical constructivist positions Silverman (1987) uses as he discusses how doctors and patients produce the reality they experience.

4. I used one version of this perspective in my earlier writings, which explored how larger structural arrangements were reflected in and reinforced by the ways doctors and patients communicated during medical encounters (Fisher 1986). In the current project I am still interested in how structural arrangements penetrate provider-patient interactions, but my focus has shifted.

5. Harding (1991:158) sees this position as the construction of scientists and scientific institutions, whom she refers to as "fast guns for hire."

6. Hartmann (1981:14), for example, depicts capitalism and patriarchy as a dual system of oppression. In so doing, she retrieves patriarchy from the purely ideological by locating it in the material realm. She argues that patriarchy is "a set of social relations between men which have a material base, and which through hierarchy, establish or create interdependence and solidarity between men that enables them to dominate women" (14). Young (1981:49) tells a slightly different story. For her, capitalism and patriarchy are a single set of analytically integrated categories. She claims that "patriarchal relations are internally related to production relations as a whole" (49).

7. In this section my discussion of Foucault is indebted to insights provided by Nancy Fraser (1989).

8. Power and resistance are the central topic of Fisher and Davis (1993), especially the introduction (Davis and Fisher 1993).

9. This is the position Fraser (1989) takes in her work.

10. Much of this section is influenced by two books that address the same moment in history; however, they do so from different theoretical positions: *The Social Transformation of American Medicine* by Paul Starr (1982), especially chapters 1–3, and *American Medicine in the Public Interest* by Rosemary Stevens (1966), especially chapters 1 and 2.

11. However, working-class women, who were described as stronger than upper-class women, could work for wages as well as reproduce. Positioning women in this way reproduced the hierarchy both between men and women and among women.

12. Although dominant beliefs may have changed over the years, both the realities of gender, race, and class and the cultural assumptions associated with these structural locations continue to play an all-too-important role in the way health care is delivered.

13. In this new kind of school, the training of nurses was extended from one to two years, and the hospital was staffed with graduate nurses rather than students (Stevens 1966).

14. As Starr (1982) points out, these same social forces contributed to the rise of labor unions, trade associations, corporations, and trusts.

15. Starr's (1982) history provides an especially interesting view of the foundational interrelationship among institutions—the hospital association, the national organization of doctors, private foundations, and the insurance industry. Although the issues may be different today, many of the players are the same, as are their practices. Shared class, gender, race, and professional interests continue to play an all-too-important role in the pursuit of policy, just as they did in the past.

16. Others—osteopathy, chiropractic, and Christian Science—remained independent and survived on their own, while those incorporated into the medical professions were largely lost (Starr 1982).

17. Starr (1982) reports that seven institutions received two-thirds of the funds.

18. The Graduate Medical Education National Advisory Committee (1979) quoted the following description of a nurse practitioner from a Department of Health, Education and Welfare report: "Today's nurse, operating in an expanded role as a professional nurse practitioner, provides direct patient care to individuals, families, and other groups in a variety of settings. . . . The nurse practitioner engages in independent decision-making about the nursing needs of clients, and collaborates with other health professionals, such as physicians, social worker, and nutritionists, in making decisions about other health care needs. The nurse working in an expanded role practices in primary, acute, and chronic health care settings. As a member of the health care team, the nurse practitioner plans and institutes health care programs" (216–217).

Although the definition of physician's assistants specifies that they work under physician supervision, the nurse practitioner is defined as a more independent, collaborative member of the team. In practice these differences are not as great as they might seem. However, they do reflect nursing's struggle for autonomy and its greater organizational coherence. For the most part, physician's assistants were at first relatively unorganized paramedics who served during the Viet Nam War.

19. I talk more about how this research could influence nursing's struggle for professional autonomy in Chapter Eight. And in the Epilogue I address the larger policy issues associated with reorganizing the health-care delivery system.

THREE *Complaints Marked as Social Psychological: The Medical Consultation*

1. From now on I refer to the nurse practitioners and the patients by their first names and to the doctors by their titles and last names. Although in so doing I reproduce the asymmetry all too prevalent in society and in the institution of medicine, this is the way providers consistently are referred to and refer to themselves and to patients. It is, therefore, an important part of the situated process of making meaning, of producing, reproducing, or undermining gendered and professional identities.

2. Back-channel comments of this kind have been found to indicate that the listener is attending to what the speaker is saying (Duncan 1972).

3. Dots indicate that the speaker's voice is trailing off.

4. Slash marks indicate an interruption.

FOUR   *Complaints Marked as Social Psychological: The Nursing Consultation*

1. Despite being told by the receptionist that Katherine was a nurse practitioner, patients often assumed she was a doctor. Her white coat and stethoscope marked her as a medical provider, and the most culturally familiar provider of medical services in our society is a doctor. In addition, Katherine was the only medical provider in the setting, and she was clearly providing rather than assisting in the provision of care. Although women are much more often nurses than doctors, under these conditions patients' persistently identified Katherine as a doctor—an identity that they marked by referring to her as "doctor" and that she consistently corrected.

2. Although by most accounts Prudence would be considered working class and Katherine certainly would not, the discussion here can be read as establishing a kind of class-based solidarity. One of the marks of the middle class, in a culture that claims to avoid most such codes, is a system of etiquette. In this system it is both inappropriate and unappealing to air one's dirty linen in public. Katherine locates Prudence as someone who does not want to talk about her private life publicly, as someone like her. In so doing she not only diminishes the distance between professional and layperson but works to establish a solidarity based on class.

FIVE   *Complaints Coded as Medical: The Medical Consultation*

1. In my experience it is often different when a woman physician walks into an examining room. Neither her white coat nor a stethoscope is enough to establish that she is the doctor. Women physicians are often assumed to be nurses and are frequently asked to establish their professional status linguistically. Commonly, women physicians introduce themselves by establishing that they are the doctor— for example, by saying, "Hello, I'm doctor so and so." Similarly, it is quite common to hear people refer to their male physicians as "doctor" but to mark the gendered exception to the norm when their physician is a woman by referring to her as a "woman doctor."

2. This medical history is part of the mental checklist that doctors use to establish a full picture of the patient's health. It usually starts at the top of the body and works down. Here, Doctor Johnson starts and stops at the head. He then moves on to a physical examination during which he continues to ask medical-history questions in a hit-or-miss fashion. I have seen this strategy used often as a time-saving measure, and it may be a useful one. But for my purposes it is too long and too unfocused to be successfully analyzed.

3. At the time I collected this data I held an adjunct appointment.

4. At the time I was collecting this data, I was forty-five, but a considerable amount of time has passed since then.

5. This use of "Daddy" is very much part of the cultural lexicon of the Southeast.

6. Syphilis, gonorrhea, and chlamydia are examples of the sexually transmitted diseases he does not screen for.

7. But he misses another medical cue. At forty-five Muriel may be experiencing some of the symptoms associated with menopause, one of which is being emotionally upset.

SIX   *Complaints Coded as Medical: The Nursing Consultation*

1. The great majority of the doctors I have observed are men. I know that situation is changing now, but it had not yet changed when I was collecting my data.

2. The exception is clinical depression. If the patient's symptoms indicate the kind of depression that can be treated medically, it is more likely to be addressed.

3. Although in the previous case I criticized Doctor Johnson for not exploring why Muriel had a hysterectomy, I do not make the same complaint against Claudia Sussen. Why not? Muriel came to the doctor seven years after her uterus had been removed. Given her presenting complaint of vaginal bleeding, it was medically important to determine why the hysterectomy had been performed in the first place, especially because cancer had such a significant place in Doctor Johnson's differential diagnosis. With Pat, there is no indication of a reproductively related problem. Claudia's response to the information that Pat had a hysterectomy seems quite appropriate. Once the topic is raised, she takes the opportunity to educate the patient about prevention.

4. I wonder about this, especially because I know something about Claudia's private life. After a bad marriage she looked for and found a man she identifies as a good man.

5. In the earlier consultations Doctor Aster and Katherine spoke from consistent, albeit different, discursive positions. So did Wendy (Doctor Aster's patient), but Prudence (Katherine's patient) did not. Prudence struggled internally over competing discourses about the appropriate way to be a woman worker in the paid labor force and a member of a nuclear family.

SEVEN   *Institutional Patterns of Interpretation*

1. Caring as a gendered activity and as a political practice will be discussed in Chapter Eight.

2. This tension is most clearly in evidence when the patient resists some aspect of the diagnosis or treatment being recommended by the provider. I address this tension more fully when I discuss the patient's resistance later in this chapter.

3. As I pointed out earlier, it is my opinion that race plays a role here as well; however, when both the provider and the patient share the unmarked dominant status, race is not visible. It seems to emerge only with a contrast. This insight

raises an important empirical question about what the production of identity and the nature of the professional relationship would be if both provider and patient shared a marked racial category.

4. Although I do not have the data to support my speculations, I suspect that the discussion of sexuality provides a site for Claudia and Pat to talk in ways that generate a sense of their common experiences as women, and the discussion of relationships does not. As a liberal, white, middle-class woman, Claudia is located in ways that facilitate her ability to relate to Pat's sexual inhibitions but hinder her ability to relate to her reservations about relationships.

5. I discuss these struggles in some detail in a later section of this chapter.

6. The topic here is a medical one. At first I wondered whether the nature of the topic produced this interaction. I concluded that it did not. Nurse practitioner and patient discuss many medical topics in this consultation, and nowhere else does this kind of interaction occur. Furthermore, the encounter is marked by Pat's successful resistance even when the topic is medical. Success in this kind of interaction is, from my observations, rare indeed. Thus, a struggle for control does not seem to be facilitated here because the topic is medical.

7. This distinction in no way minimizes the intrusion of social/ideological discourses into topics that are presumably medical in nature.

8. It is part of the common lore that women's medical complaints often get trivialized. When I talk about my earlier research about doctors and women patients (Fisher 1986), women are forever telling me horror stories. For example, in my graduate school days, a fellow student went to the emergency room complaining of extreme pain in the lower right quadrant of her abdomen. She was told it was nerves, and tranquilizers were prescribed. It was an ectopic pregnancy, and she nearly lost her life. Unfortunately, this is not an unusual story. I have been told about ulcers undiagnosed and heart conditions untreated. The evidence is not all circumstantial. Even the National Institutes of Health have recognized this problem by organizing a special section to fund research about women's health risks.

9. Perhaps this insistence on medical topics is one of the ways the differences in presenting complaints—social psychological and medical—are manifested. However, this emphasis on medical topics does not occur in the nursing consultation even when the presenting complaint is easily seen as medical.

10. When Wendy hears, or thinks she hears, that her decision to seek medical advice is being trivialized, she responds in a similar manner. She tells the doctor that it was her husband's idea that she come to see him. In this way, she too reproduces the very discursive position she has been resisting.

11. As everyday speakers of English, we mark the nondominant category, making distinctions all too clear. When we refer to women physicians and women lawyers, we are signaling more than gender. We are marking the deviation from the norm. Similarly, when we refer to a male nurse, we are also marking these distinctions, but there is a difference. The way we mark these categories also implies value. Referring to women doctors and lawyers signals a move to more valued positions; referring to male nurses signals quite the opposite (compare Lakoff 1973).

12. I have some further validation for this supposition. After my work in the

model family-practice clinic a student of mine observed the same doctors delivering care to men patients, and the process was different. Men were differentiated by class and race, with deference being given to higher-status men (Groce 1986).

EIGHT *The Politics of Location*

1. The analysis in this section appeared in a slightly different form in previous papers (Fisher 1991, 1993).

2. Whether providers and patients can both speak in a medical voice is still an open empirical question; however, prior work suggests that at least for doctors and patients there is not a shared capacity for medical talk. Patients' abilities to enter the domain marked as medical varies by gender and is probably influenced as well by other factors such as race, class, and professional status (Fisher and Groce 1990).

3. Hall, like Silverman (1987), Fraser (1989), Harding (1991), and Haraway (1991), is relying on Foucauldian postmodernism and poststructuralism and like most of these scholars (except Silverman) is looking for a way to combine them with more structural insights.

4. The internal debates about nursing as a profession make this lack of cohesion all too clear. If education and credentials define the profession and stratify the practitioners, then the practitioners who by education and credentials are defined as the professionals become the political actors, and they are divided from others. These divisions take several forms—academic nurses and clinicians, nurse practitioners and registered nurses, registered nurses, and licensed vocational nurses, and nurses and other hospital workers. Although these factions then fight among themselves, doctors continue to sit on nursing boards and are able to manipulate the factions in ways that all too often preserve the interests of doctors and keep nurses in their place as marginalized and subordinate workers fighting for professional recognition.

5. Although historically medicine has predominantly accepted male practitioners and nursing has accepted females practitioners, that has been changing. Increasingly, women are entering medicine, and men are becoming nurses. But changing the gender of the practitioner does not automatically change the gendered nature of the profession. Quite the contrary. At least at this time medicine continues to be gendered male. It is characterized by a war discourse: doctors do battle against disease. Nursing, by contrast, remains gendered female. It is characterized by a discourse of nurturance: what differentiates medicine from nursing, according to nurses, is that nurses care and doctors do not.

6. In fact, this is the conclusion I reach in Fisher (1986).

7. Here, I am talking about something quite different from whether nurses should be trained to substitute for doctors or to do something different like wellness care. I am talking about the ways nurses locate themselves in a political discourse.

EPILOGUE *Making Health-Care Policy*

1. In the nursing literature the argument is usually framed in terms of substitutability or alternatives. Should nurse practitioners be trained to do medical diagnosis and treatment like family-practice doctors, or should they do something different like education, prevention, wellness care, or healing touch? I am both entering and reframing this debate.

2. The experience in Holland suggests that 85 percent of all births are normal and can be handled effectively by midwives.

REFERENCES

Arditti, R., P. Brennan, and S. Cavarak, eds. 1980. *Science and Liberation*. Boston: South End Press.

Arney, W., and B. Bergen. 1983. The Chronic Patient. *Sociology of Health and Illness* 5 (1):1–24.

Bartky, S. L. 1988. Foucault, Femininity, and the Modernization of Patriarchal Power. In *Feminism and Foucault: Reflections on Resistance*, ed. I. Diamond and L. Quinby, 61–86. Boston: Northeastern University Press.

Bordo, S. 1988. Anorexia Nervosa: Psychopathology as the Crystallization of Culture. In *Feminism and Foucault: Reflections on Resistance*, ed. I. Diamond and L. Quinby, 87–118. Boston: Northeastern University Press.

Brown, C. 1981. Mothers, Fathers and Children: From Private to Public Patriarchy. In *Women and Revolution: A Discussion of the Unhappy Marriage of Marxism and Feminism*, ed. L. Sargent, 239–268. Boston: South End Press.

Brown, E. R. 1979. *Rockefeller Medicine Men: Medicine and Capitalism in the Progressive Era*. Berkeley: University of California Press.

Brown, R. 1965. *Social Psychology*. Glencoe, Ill.: Free Press.

Butler, J. 1990. *Gender Trouble: Feminism and the Subversion of Identity*. New York: Routledge.

Cicourel, A. V. 1964. *Method and Measurement in Sociology*. New York: Free Press.

Cott, N. F. 1977. *The Bonds of Womanhood*. New Haven: Yale University Press.

Crowley, A. E., and S. I. Etzel, and E. S. Petersen. 1984. Undergraduate Medical Education. *Journal of the American Medical Association* 252:1525.

Davis, K. 1988. *Power under the Microscope: Toward a Grounded Theory of Gender Relations in Medical Encounters*. Rotterdam: Foris

———. 1994. *Re-making the Female Body*. New York: Routledge.

Davis, K., and S. Fisher. 1993. Power and the Female Subject. In *Negotiating at the Margins: The Gendered Discourses of Power and Resistance*, ed. S. Fisher and K. Davis, 3–20. New Brunswick, N.J.: Rutgers University Press.

Diers, D., and S. Molde. 1979. Some Conceptual and Methodological Issues in Nurse Practitioner Research. *Nursing and Health* 2 (March): 73–84.

Duncan, S., Jr. 1972. Some Signals and Rules for Taking Speaking Turns in Conversation. *Journal of Personality and Social Psychology* 23:283–292.

Eastaugh, S. E. 1981. An Efficient Solution to Primary Care Maldistribution. *Hospital Progress* 62:32.

Ehrenreich, B., and D. English. 1972. *Witches, Midwives and Nurses: A History of Women Healers*. Glass Mountain Pamphlet 1. Brooklyn, N.Y.: Feminist Press.

————. 1973. *Complaints and Disorders: The Sexual Politics of Sickness.* Glass Mountain Pamphlet 2. Brooklyn, N.Y.: Feminist Press.

————. 1979. *For Her Own Good.* Garden City, N.Y.: Doubleday, Anchor.

Eisenberg, D. M., R. C. Kessler, C. Foster, S. E. Norloc, D. R. Calkins, and T. L. Delbanco. 1993. Unconventional Medicine in the United States. *New England Journal of Medicine* 328(4):246–252.

Fisher, S. 1986. *In the Patient's Best Interest: Women and the Politics of Medical Decisions.* New Brunswick, N.J.: Rutgers University Press.

————. 1991. A Discourse of the Social: Medical Talk/Power Talk/Oppositional Talk? *Discourse and Society* 2(2):157–182.

————. 1993. Gender, Power, Resistance: Is Care the Remedy? In *Negotiating at the Margins: The Gendered Discourses of Power and Resistance*, ed. S. Fisher and K. Davis, 87–121. New Brunswick, N.J.: Rutgers University Press.

Fisher, S., and K. Davis, eds. 1993. *Negotiating at the Margins: The Gendered Discourses of Power and Resistance.* New Brunswick, N.J.: Rutgers University Press.

Fisher, S., and S. Groce. 1990. Accounting Practices in Medical Interviews. *Language in Society* 19(June):225–250.

Fisher, S., and A. D. Todd. 1986. Friendly Persuasion: Negotiating Decisions to Use Oral Contraceptives. In *Discourse and Institutional Authority: Medicine, Education, and Law*, ed. S. Fisher, and A. D. Todd, 3–25. Norwood, N.J.: Ablex.

Foucault, M. 1978. *The History of Sexuality, 1: An Introduction.* Trans. R. Hurley. New York: Pantheon.

————. 1979. *Discipline and Punish: The Birth of the Prison.* Trans. A. Sheridan. New York: Random House, Vintage.

————. 1981. Questions of Method. *Ideology and Consciousness* 8(Spring):3–14.

Fraser, N. 1989. *Unruly Practices: Power, Discourse and Gender in Contemporary Social Theory.* Minneapolis: University of Minnesota Press.

Freidson, E. 1970. *Profession of Medicine.* New York: Dodd, Mead.

Gleeson, S. n.d. Nurses for National Health Care. Unpublished position paper.

Goffman, E. 1956. The Nature of Difference and Demeanor. *American Anthropologist* 58:473–502.

Gordon, L. 1988. *Heroes of Their Own Lives: The Politics and History of Family Violence, Boston, 1860–1980.* New York: Viking Penguin.

Graduate Medical Education National Advisory Committee. 1979. *Interim Report of the Graduate Medical Education National Advisory Committee to the Secretary.* Washington, D.C.: Department of Health, Education and Welfare.

————. 1980. *GMENAC Summary Report to the Secretary, U.S. Department of Health and Human Services.* Washington, D.C.: Department of Health and Human Services.

Graham, H. 1985. Provider, Negotiations and Mediators: Women as Hidden Care Givers. In *Women, Health and Healing*, ed. E. Lewin and V. Olesen, 25–52. New York: Tavistock.

Gramsci, A. 1971. *Selections from the Prison Notebooks.* New York: International Publishers.

Groce, S. B., 1986. Medical Interviews, Treatment Decisions and the Social Construction of Reality: An Analysis of Doctor-Patient Communication. Ph.D. diss., University of Tennessee, Knoxville.

Grossberg, L. 1986. On Postmodernism and Articulation: An Interview with Stuart Hall. *Journal of Communications Inquiry* 10(2):45–60.

Hall, S. 1986. The Problem of Ideology—Marxism without Guarantees. *Journal of Communications Inquiry* 10(2):28–44.

Haraway, D. J. 1991. *Simians, Cyborgs and Women: The Reinventing of Nature*. New York: Routledge.

Harding, S. 1986. *The Science Question in Feminism*. Ithaca, N.Y.: Cornell University Press.

———. 1991. *Whose Science? Whose Knowledge?: Thinking from Women's Lives*. Ithaca, N.Y.: Cornell University Press.

Hartmann, H. 1981. The Unhappy Marriage of Marxism and Feminism: Towards a More Progressive Union. In *Women and Revolution: A Discussion of the Unhappy Marriage of Marxism and Feminism*, ed. L. Sargent, 1–42. Boston: South End Press.

Hartsock, N. 1983. *Money, Sex and Power*. Boston: Longman.

Henley, N. 1975. Power, Sex and Nonverbal Communication. In *Language and Sex: Difference and Dominance*, ed. B. Thorne and N. Henley, 184–202. Rowley, Mass.: Newbury House.

Jourard, S. M., and P. Lasakow. 1958. Some Factors in Self Disclosure. *Journal of Abnormal and Social Psychology* 56:91–98.

Knorr-Cetina, K., and A. V. Cicourel, eds. 1981. *Advances in Social Theory and Methodology: Toward and Integration of Micro- and Macro-sociologies*. Boston: Routledge & Kegan Paul.

Kuhn, T. S. 1962. *The Structure of Scientific Revolutions*. Chicago: University of Chicago Press.

Lakoff, R. 1973. *Language and Woman's Place*. New York: Harper, Colophon.

Latour, B., and S. Woolgar. 1979. *Laboratory Life: The Social Construction of Fact*. Beverly Hills, Calif.: Sage.

Lohr, K. N., and R. H. Brooks. 1984. Quality Assurance in Medicine. *American Behavioral Scientist* 27:583.

Lynaugh, J. E., and C. M. Fagin. 1988. Nursing Comes of Age. *Image: Journal of Nursing Scholarship* 20(4):184–190.

MacKinnon, C. 1987. *Feminism Unmodified: Discourses on Life and Law*. Cambridge: Harvard University Press.

Martin, B. 1988. Feminism, Criticism and Foucault. In *Feminism and Foucault: Reflections on Resistance*, ed. I. Diamond and L. Quinby, 3–20. Boston: Northeastern University Press.

Mehan, H. 1979. *Learning Lessons: Social Organization in the Classroom*. Cambridge: Harvard University Press.

Mehan, H., and L. Wood. 1975. *The Reality of Ethnomethodology*. New York: Wiley.

Melosh, B. 1982. *The Physician's Hand*. Philadelphia: Temple University Press.

Mishler, E. G. 1984. *The Discourse of Medicine: Dialectics of Medical Interviews*. Norwood, N.J.: Ablex.

Morris, S. B., and D. B. Smith. 1977. The Distribution of Physician Extenders. *Medical Care* 15:1045.

Prather, J. 1990. Why Women Use Tranquilizers. In *Drug Use: A Sourcebook of Patterns and Factors*, ed. B. Forster and J. C. Salloway, 303–318. Lewiston, N.Y.: Edwin Mellen Press.

Prather, J., and L. S. Fidell. 1973. Sex Differences in the Context and Style of Medical Advertisements. *Social Science and Medicine* 9:23–26.

Reverby, S. M. 1987. *Ordered to Care: The Dilemma of American Nursing*. Cambridge, England: Cambridge University Press.

Riessman, C. K. 1983. Women and Medicalization. *Social Policy* 14:3–18.

Riley, D. 1988. *"Am I That Name?" Feminism and the Category of "Women" in History*. Minneapolis: University of Minnesota Press.

Roueché, B. 1977. *Together: A Casebook of Joint Practices in Primary Care*. Chicago: National Joint Practice Commission.

Rouse, J. 1987. *Knowledge and Power: Toward a Political Philosophy of Science*. Ithaca, N.Y.: Cornell University Press.

———. 1991. The Dynamics of Power and Knowledge in Science. *Journal of Philosophy* 22:658–665.

Ruby, G. 1981. New Health Professionals in Child and Maternal Care. In *Better Health for Our Children: A National Strategy, Report of the Select Panel for the Promotion of Child Health, IV*. Publication 79-55071. Washington, D.C.: Public Health Service, Department of Health and Human Services.

Sacket, D. L., W. O. Spitzer, M. Gent, and R. S. Roberts. 1974. The Burlington Randomized Trial of the Nurse Practitioner: Health Outcomes of Patients. *Annals of Internal Medicine* 80(2)(February):137–142.

Scott, J. W. 1988. *Gender and the Politics of History*. New York: Columbia University Press.

Shamansky, S. L. 1985. Nurse Practitioner and Primary Care Research: Promises and Pitfalls. In *Annual Review of Nursing Research*, ed. H. Werley and J. Fitzpatric, vol. 3, 107–125. New York: Springer.

Silverman, D. 1987. *Communication and Medical Practice: Social Relations in the Clinic*. London: Sage.

Silverman, D., and B. Torode B. 1980. *The Material World: Theories of Language and Its Limits*. London: Routledge & Kegan Paul.

Smoyak, S. A. 1977. Problems in Interprofessional Relations. *Bulletin of the New York Academy of Medicine* 53(1):51–59.

Starr, P. 1982. *The Social Transformation of American Medicine*. New York: Basic Books.

Stevens, R. 1966. *American Medicine in the Public Interest*. New Haven: Yale University Press.

Tarlov, A. R. 1983. Shattuck Lecture—The Increasing Supply of Physicians, the Changing Structure of the Health Service System, and the Future Practice of Medicine. *New England Journal of Medicine* 308:1235.

Todd, A. D. 1989. *Intimate Adversaries: Cultural Conflicts between Doctors and Women Patients*. Philadelphia: University of Pennsylvania Press.

Toronto, J. C. 1989. What Can Feminists Learn about Morality from Caring? In *Gender, Body and Knowledge: Feminist Reconstructions of Being and Knowing*, ed. A. M. Jaggar and S. Bordo, 172–187. New Brunswick, N.J.: Rutgers University Press.

Volosinov, V. 1973. *Marxism and the Philosophy of Language*. New York: Seminar Press.

Waitzkin, H. B. 1983. *The Second Sickness: Contradictions in Capitalist Health Care*. New York: Free Press.

Waitzkin, H. B., and B. Waterman. 1974. *The Exploitation of Illness in Capitalist Societies*. Indianapolis: Bobbs-Merrill.

Wartenburg, T. 1990. *From Domination to Transformation*. Philadelphia: Temple University Press.

Young, I. 1981. Beyond the Unhappy Marriage: A Critique of the Dual System Theory. In *Women and Revolution: A Discussion of the Unhappy Marriage of Marxism and Feminism*, ed. L. Sargent, 43–70. Boston: South End Press.

INDEX

ABOUT THE AUTHOR

Sue Fisher is a professor at Wesleyan University, where she teaches in the sociology department as well as in the Science in Society and Women's Studies Programs. She is author of a number of related books, including *In the Patient's Best Interest: Women and the Politics of Medical Decisions*; she is coeditor (with K. Davis) of *Negotiating at the Margins: The Gendered Discourse of Power and Resistance*.